AGENT OF MERCY

THE UNTOLD STORY OF,
DR. ARCHIBALD S. MAXWELL,
CIVIL WAR SURGEON & IOWA STATE SANITARY AGENT

BY GEORGE C. MAXWELL

Olga and Steve, Merry Christmas! I treasure your friendship. George Maxwell 2015

Library of Congress Control Number:2015918456
CreateSpace Independent Publishing Platform, North Charleston, SC

Library of Congress Cataloging In Publication Data

Maxwell, George Collier
Agent of Mercy: The Untold Story of Dr. Archibald S. Maxwell Civil War Surgeon & Iowa State Sanitary Agent

Includes bibliographical references.
ISBN-13: 978-1519120304
ISBN-10: 151920303

To my wife and children

TABLE OF CONTENTS

INTRODUCTION

This book is about Dr. Archibald S. Maxwell. He is my great-great-great grandfather, and he was a surgeon in the Civil War. The corpus of this history is based on letters and reports that he wrote or that were written about him. Some of these letters were published in the local newspaper in Davenport during the Civil War, and others were archived in Iowa State Records. This book sets his actions and activities in the context of the Iowa Sanitary Affairs/Soldiers' Relief efforts in which he participated during the Civil War. Sanitary affairs were in many instances combined with soldiers' relief. These efforts in Iowa took on more than a whiff of the political caused by competition between the two rival Iowa sanitary organizations from 1861 to the end of 1863. Archibald was drawn into that rivalry as a supporter of Annie Wittenmyer.

My efforts to discover the facts surrounding his Civil War service began in front of a white tag board with an enlarged copy of Archibald's 1884 obituary at a Maxwell family reunion in Scott County, Iowa. The reunion took place an easy drive from Davenport, Iowa, where Archibald lived and practiced before and after his service in the Civil War.

After the Maxwell reunion, I took several trips to the State Historical Society of Iowa in Des Moines, Iowa, to see what they might have. The account in this book finds its roots in the letters, newspaper articles, and books that I discovered there. These sources reveal a rich tapestry of benevolent work by many men and women across the North (particularly in Iowa), including Archibald. They labored on the home front. They risked life and health with the army in the field to provide the brave soldiers, broken and sick in the cause of preserving the Union, with better care, which the army found itself unable to do. His thread in this tapestry touched and crossed many other people important in Iowa sanitary affairs—Annie Wittenmyer, Colonel Ira Gifford, Governor Samuel J. Kirkwood, and Annie Wittenmyer's nemesis, the Reverend A. J. Kynett, to name a few.

In fact, I was most surprised to learn of the level of intrigue and political gamesmanship that occurred between the two groups competing to meet Iowa troops' medical assistance needs. Archibald supported Mrs. Annie Wittenmyer, who was The Iowa State Sanitary Agent by special Iowa law. Reverend A. J. Kynett and his organization attempted at every turn to discredit her and ultimately to deprive her of the donations of the medical assistance that she needed to sustain her organization in the field.

In the course of my research, I learned that Archibald served his country and the state of Iowa in many medical capacities. In two short years, 1862–63, he wore many hats. He was a member of the Scott County Soldiers Relief Association, a Surgeon in various capacities at the front, Military Hospital Assistant Surgeon in Keokuk, Iowa and Professor of Physiology and Pathology at the Physicians and Surgeons College in Keokuk, Iowa. Finally, he served as an Iowa state sanitary agent along with Iowa State Sanitary Agent Annie Wittenmyer. He supported her efforts to provide much-needed assistance to the wounded and sick Union soldiers in the Civil War's Western Theater hospitals. Archibald was present in the aftermath of the battles at Fort Donelson, Shiloh, Corinth, Iuka, Helena, and Vicksburg, tending the sick and wounded, delivering desperately needed medical and nutritional supplies, and helping the soldiers to get home.

You will note that I refer to him as Archibald throughout the text. He often called himself by his initials, A.S. Others called him just Dr. Maxwell. I have chosen to call him, Archibald and mean no disrespect to his position as a surgeon and doctor. Archibald is my great-great-great grandfather. If my address seems familiar, it is to convey the sense of connection between us. While it is probably easier to be objective about him and his actions given that over 150 years separate his birth and mine, he is my relative. If the reader wants a completely unbiased account, the individual will likely have to search elsewhere.

One more important note: Medical assistance for soldiers in Archibald's day during the Civil War was quite different from today. While the U.S. military had a corps of surgeons at the beginning of the war, it was not staffed, supplied, or prepared to provide the amount and kind of medical attention that the sick and wounded volunteer soldiers needed. Because the Army was incapable of providing that level of medical assistance, public-private benevolent organizations, the largest of which was the U.S. Sanitary Commission, arose to address these sanitary affairs, which is how they referred to the medical assistance in that day. "Sanitary affairs" and sanitary goods included basic medical supplies, nutritious food, nursing, doctoring and surgery, and other medical assistance. The larger organizations were public in the sense that the commissioners who ran them were appointed by public officials, but private in the sense that the funding sources for much of their efforts came from private donations of goods and money.

Because of the sacrifices of Union soldiers and those who provided medical assistance to them, Lincoln's words in his Gettysburg address continue to be true today, "the nation conceived in Liberty and dedicated to the proposition that all men are created equal" did not perish and remained "a government of the people, by the people, for the people." We owe it to the memory of those Union soldiers to recall their sacrifices and to meet the challenges of our generation so that Lincoln's words continue to ring true for future generations.

While there are certainly books that address individual surgeons' accounts, Dr. Archibald S. Maxwell, was different because he was more than just a surgeon, and the other roles he played had a political dimension to them. However, if in search of other books on Civil War surgeons, you could start with *Personal Memoirs of John H. Brinton, Major and Surgeon U.S.V., 1861–1865* by John H. Brinton. More recent efforts to publish the letters and journals include (1) *Letters of Civil War Surgeon* edited by Paul Fatout (Purdue Research Foundation 1996); (2) *Letters from a Civil War Surgeon: The Letters of Dr. William Child of the 5th New Hampshire Volunteers* by William Child (Polar Bear and Co. 2001); (3) *The Journal of a Civil War Surgeon/J. Franklin Dryer*, Edited by Michael B. Chesson (University of Nebraska Press 2003); and (4) *A Surgeon's Civil War The Letters and Diary of Daniel M. Holt, M.D.* Edited by James M. Greiner, Janet L Coryell; and James Smither (The Kent State University Press 1994). These each provide an account by an individual surgeon, usually presented by an editor that has organized a series of letters or diary entries.

This book attempts to chronicle Archibald's service based on letters and reports written by Archibald himself as well as others who travelled with him. It also attempts to explain his role in the larger context. The book, however, is not meant to be an in-depth study of anything beyond the role Archibald played. It is not meant to be a commentary on Civil War medicine. While it does mention the political environment surrounding Iowa sanitary affairs, Annie Wittenmyer, and the U.S. Sanitary Commission, it only addresses these topics as necessary to explain Archibald's role that he played in certain events. For works on these related topics, please see footnote one. [1]

With regard to his letters, I have tried to maintain a light touch in the editing to keep his words or the words of the speaker. If, however, for grammar or understanding it was necessary to insert or replace a word or insert punctuation, I have done so. If I inserted or replaced a word [for clarity], I paced square brackets around the word.

I hope you have as much fun reading the book as I had researching and writing it.

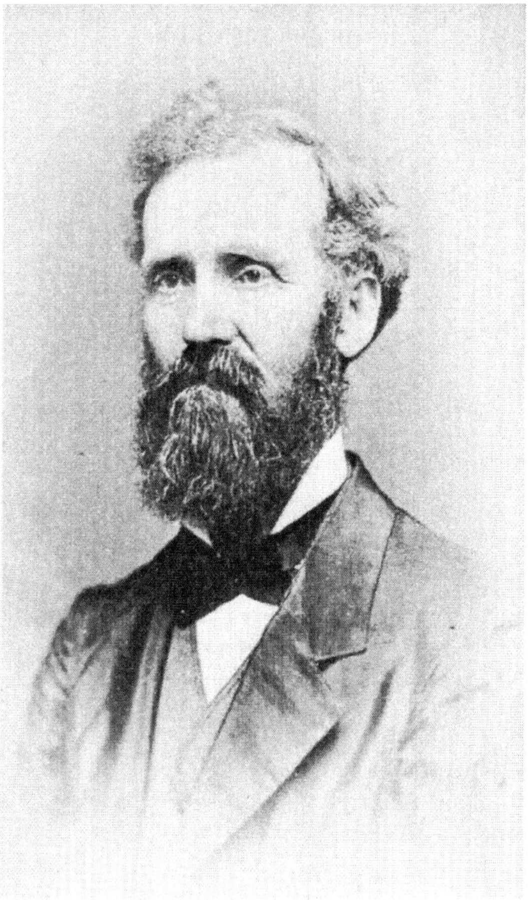

Dr. Archibald S. Maxwell

PROLOGUE:
The Call for Medical Assistance Becomes Clear in the West

It began with a train on an August night in 1861. That night train pulled into the 14th Street station in St. Louis, Missouri, filled with 100 groaning, wounded Union soldiers.[2] These one hundred brave, not quite green, Union volunteers had been wounded in a losing effort on a field many miles to the southwest of St. Louis near Springfield, Missouri. The lost battle would be called Wilson's Creek and remembered by some as the Western Theater's Bull Run. On this August night and ever after, it would become abundantly clear to many that the U.S. Army had failed their wounded warriors in incomprehensible ways. However, the people, including my ancestor, Dr. Archibald Maxwell, did not fail them, but volunteered in sanitary commissions and soldiers' relief organizations to provide the medical assistance to help the sick and wounded Union warriors.

The Confederate and Union soldiers fought the Battle of Wilson's Creek on August 10, 1861. On that day, the 100, wounded soldiers on that night train, along with 5,100 other brave Union brothers, stood against repeated attacks by 15,000 Confederate soldiers until their leader, Union General Lyon, was shot dead. In the battle, 721 Union soldiers were wounded, and an additional 241 died. These hundred wounded along with 621 other wounded brothers endured a grueling, 120-mile retreat with the remainder of the Union Army to Rolla, Missouri, over rutted dirt roads in horse drawn ambulances and army wagons with only "limited food and water."[3] At Rolla, the Army loaded 100 of those wounded on the night train bound for St. Louis, with no food provisioned for the 10-hour journey.

Upon arrival that night in St. Louis, the wounded Union soldiers were transported in furniture carts three miles to the New House of Refuge Hospital that the Army had opened on August 6th and staffed with two surgeons and one doctor. When the 100 wounded arrived, "bare walls, bare floors, and an empty kitchen received them."[4] The new army hospital had no beds, no bedsteads, no stoves, no bedding, no food, and no nurses. In short, nothing prepared. In these deplorable conditions, the wounded slept on "hard boards." Over the course of the week, three or four hundred wounded comrades in arms joined the first hundred.

The starving soldiers were fed on the night of their arrival, but not by the Army. The people of St. Louis fed the wounded. The civilians in the neighborhood near the hospital brought over cooked food to feed the hungry "shattered and travel-worn" wounded.

The Army's incompetence did not go unnoticed. A group of concerned St. Louis citizens formed the Western Sanitary Commission to provide the medical supplies and care that the Army could not. On September 5th, Major General Fremont issued an order that appointed commissioners and set out the parameters under which the Western Sanitary Commission could work to ameliorate the military medical corps' deficiencies. It was not until more than a year later, in December 1862, that the War Department ratified General Fremont's earlier order.[5]

While the Western Sanitary Commission claimed that things at the hospital improved in the first few weeks, the descriptions they provided make that difficult to believe. Their report recorded that "many of the badly wounded men lay in the hospital" still wearing the same soiled, bloodstained uniform "in which they had been brought from the battlefield three weeks before."[6] The wounded slept in soiled uniforms saturated with their own blood, because the Army did not have the "necessary hospital clothing" to substitute. In fact, "the wounds of many had not been dressed since the first dressing after battle; others were still suffering from un-extracted bullets and pieces of shell."[7]

The disastrous circumstances in St. Louis that greeted the wounded of the Battle of Wilson's Creek and other battles like it made clear to the people in the western states, like my ancestor, Dr. Archibald Maxwell, Governor Samuel Kirkwood of Iowa, and others that the U.S. Army could not be trusted to take care of the thousands of citizens who had recently volunteered to save the Union. After all, the Iowa 1st Regiment had fought with distinction at the Battle of Wilson's Creek and suffered 141 wounded, making this disaster very personal to Iowans. Incidents like the empty hospital in St. Louis lay bare that the Army Medical Corps was woefully unprepared to provide even the limited medical assistance available at that time. Even by those standards, no good excuse existed to explain the Army's inability to anticipate problems and resolve the supply logistics for ensuring that its sick and wounded had beds, pillows, hospital gowns, adequate supplies of medicine, and food that could be fed a sick man. Additionally, there was no excuse for not supplying more-or-less healthy soldiers with adequate supplies of vegetables and fruit in order to prevent nutritional deficiency diseases such as scurvy. Because the Army and Army Medical Corps could not, groups such as the U.S. Sanitary Commission, Western Sanitary Commission, and Iowa Sanitary Commission—where my ancestor, Archibald, would play his part—arose to fill the gap caused by the army and Army Medical Corps' failure.

Although not mentioned in the Western Sanitary Commission's report directly, the U.S. Sanitary Commission—the private group that was supposed to coordinate providing medical assistance for the whole country—also was not present in St. Louis in August 1861 when this medical disaster unfolded before the eyes of many. The U.S. Sanitary Commission in early 1861 focused much of its efforts on the Eastern Theater and only sent its Western Theater Agent, Dr. Newberry west of the Appalachian Mountains, in mid-September 1861.[8] The sense that the Western states at first had been left to address the army's incompetence on their own appears to have fueled the creation of rival sanitary commissions, like the Western Sanitary Commission, and other homegrown solutions such as the Iowa Sanitary Commission's efforts in which Archibald would play a significant part.

These sanitary commissions and their local soldiers' relief and ladies aid societies became a major movement in the U.S. Civil War because the public demanded better medical care for its wounded and sick soldiers than the army was capable of providing, particularly at the beginning of the Civil War. The U.S. Civil War mortality rates of two out of three deaths due to disease were better than the U.S.-Mexican War rates of seven deaths from disease for every death in battle. However, by the start of the Civil War, times and circumstances had changed.[9] Communication and transportation between the war front and home had improved, enabling people at home to learn of the deplorable conditions and to make prompt responses to provide medical aid and saves lives. Archibald played his part in providing that assistance.

CHAPTER 1:
From Ohio Farm Boy to Iowa Doctor

Like the train in 1861, beginnings are important. Archibald's actions and decisions in the crucial war years can best be understood in their full context of his life up to that point. Thankfully, my ancestor left an autobiographical summary that with helpful hints that led to other sources providing a more complete picture of his pre-Civil War life.

Dr. Archibald Stephens Maxwell stood out among his brothers and sisters. While none of his older siblings sought an education or a profession, he possessed a drive, passion, and ambition to seek an education, find a profession, and achieve recognition and fortune. He found a profession, although not the one that he wanted. He achieved recognition in his field as a talented, experienced, able, and relentless surgeon and doctor. At the same time, some of his greatest contributions in the Civil War have gone relatively unnoticed. Throughout his life, he overcame obstacles with endurance and perseverance in the face of challenging and life altering events. There were moments when he could have packed up to head home, but he did not. He instead persisted onward when adversity struck in business, on the home front, in his profession, and also while serving his country during the Civil War.

Family was important to Archibald. While he was absent for extended periods, he returned, and he reached out to lift his family members up. He helped a younger brother enter the medical profession. He returned to try to save a beloved sister and also to spend the final days with a dying brother. He saved a sick brother-in-law.

Archibald was born into a frontier farming family in Tuscarawas County, Ohio, on June 23, 1818. He was the tenth of eleven children of John Maxwell and Ruth Cypherd.[10] His father, John, was a veteran of the American Revolutionary War. Archibald's parents left York County, Pennsylvania, for Ohio where land was cheaper, because his father's inheritance was insufficient to purchase land that might provide a living in Pennsylvania.[11]

Archibald's parents took their time making the trek to Tuscarawas County, Ohio. They left Pennsylvania sometime after the sale and division of John's father's estate in 1801. They stopped in Brooke County, Virginia, in 1804 (now West Virginia), where Archibald's sister, Margaret, was born. In 1806, they purchased a farm in Jefferson County, Ohio, a county on the Ohio border with West Virginia.[12] By 1811, the family had moved from Jefferson County to settle a farm in Tuscarawas County, where Archibald was born along with four of his brothers.[13]

Archibald was barely four years old when tragedy struck his family- his father died in 1822. Of John and Ruth's eleven children, Ruth had seven children under the age of 18, including a baby, David, at John's death. Of Ruth's adult children, only Jane and Margaret remained at home in 1822. The eldest son, Sam, had ventured out several years before, and the other adult daughter, Mary, was married and gone.

Two years after John's death, his daughter Margaret married and moved to Berlin in Holmes County, Ohio. [14] At the same time, Ruth left the farm in Tuscarawas County and moved her minor children, including Archibald, to Berlin, Holmes County, Ohio, too. Ruth very likely moved with her younger children to live near or with Margaret and her new husband because Ruth needed help raising the young children.[15]

As he grew up on the farm in Holmes County, Archibald hungered for knowledge and opportunity that a farm life could not provide. He attended district school where he learned the basics, but the family did not possess the means to provide an education at an academy or a college. In 1834 at the age of 16, he left the farm to apprentice as a printer.[16] In 1836 at the age of 18, he and his employer, Jacob Rosenberg, left Holmes County, Ohio, for the frontier town of Findlay, Ohio, in Western Ohio. In Findlay, Jacob Rosenberg founded the *Findlay Courier* with Archibald as his printer.

The *Findlay Courier* was a newspaper that openly supported the Democratic Party's Jacksonian politics, the politics of the outgoing President, Andrew Jackson.[17] At the time of the paper's founding, Andrew Jackson was wrapping up his second term in office, and the campaign to elect his successor was in full swing. The Democratic Party had nominated President Jackson's vice president, Martin Van Buren, for 1836 Presidential ticket. President Andrew Jackson was viewed as a champion for the common man and an opponent of the Second Bank of the United States, which President Jackson successfully eliminated by vetoing its charter.[18]

The success of the Democratic Party in electing its candidate Martin Van Buren as President in 1836 did not transfer to the *Findlay Courier* in Findlay. In November 1837, the *Findlay Courier* closed, putting Archibald out of work.[19] At the young age of 19, Archibald faced a choice. He could have returned home to Holmes County. Instead, Archibald recognized an opportunity and seized it, even though it involved working for an organization that supported political opinions he opposed.

Archibald's opportunity was to work as a foreman for a paper that supported the Whig Party, the *Hancock Republican* in Findlay. The Whig Party opposed everything about Andrew Jackson and the Democratic Party. The *Hancock Republican* began publication in February 1838 about 3 months after the demise of the *Findlay Courier*.[20] Archibald did not like the paper's politics, as appears evident from his description in his later, short autobiography. Nevertheless, he and the editor of the Whig paper, Mr. A. F. Miriam, Esq., became friends while he worked at the paper. Mr. Miriam and his wife schooled Archibald in Latin, Greek and French during the year he worked for them. He remembered them fondly forty years later with much gratitude, even if he held little regard for their politics.[21] This ability to bridge divides and differences would be a helpful trait later in life as well.

In 1839, at 21 years of age, Archibald left Findlay and moved to Mansfield, Ohio. Whether his move was triggered by his mother Ruth's death that year is unclear. In Mansfield, he joined forces with John Meredith to found the partnership of Meredith & Maxwell. The partnership published the *Shield and Banner*, a weekly Democratic newspaper in Mansfield, Richland County, Ohio, from 1839 to April 22, 1841. Archibald Maxwell and John Meredith's paper was a partisan political newspaper in support of the Democratic Party. The paper sought to "[advance] the cause of Jeffersonian democracy."[22] It was the opposite of the Whig *Hancock Republican*. As John Meredith would explain, he and A. S. Maxwell never desired to conceal "from the public [their] political predilections and attachment to Democratic principles and measures, the success of which [they deemed] essential to the perpetuation of our Republican institutions and inseparably blended with the dearest interests of the toiling millions." Archibald and John endeavored each week to "publish to the world a clear, concise, and unvarnished exhibit of democratic principles and measures and to expose promptly so far as it has been in [their] power, the schemes and machinations of opposing factions—the aristocratic few, whose object is power and money, and to obtain which [the aristocratic few] will resort to any means however disingenuous, wholly regardless of the rights and interests of the great body of the people." [23]

Mansfield in Archibald's time was a growing city filled with many talented lawyers who would leave their mark on the West. The talented bar included Samuel J. Kirkwood, Iowa's future governor and senator, and Jacob Brinkerhoff, Richland County Prosecutor, future Democratic U.S. congressman in 1842 and Ohio Supreme Court justice.[24] Archibald wanted to join their ranks. While a partner in Meredith & Maxwell, A. S. Maxwell began studying law in the office of Jacob Brinkerhoff. [25]

His study of the law led him to transition out of the newspaper business. The sale of the paper in April 1841 finally provided Archibald with the opportunity to fulfill one of his passions—a proper education. Archibald used the proceeds from the sale of newspaper to attend the Ashland Academy in Ashland, Ohio.[26] While he had wanted to go to Athens University farther away, he needed to be near Mansfield to wrap up the partnership affairs, and chose to attend the Academy in Ashland instead. He completed the Academy with honors in 18 months. Upon graduation, he continued his study of the law and pursued the beginnings of a career in politics.

Archibald was an ambitious young Democrat angling for a political position. He supported a part of the Democratic Party faction that favored limits on the expansion of slavery called the Free-Soil democrats.[27] At this time in his life, Archibald felt that many doors of possibilities were open to him, that he had joined the educated few, and that his star was bright and on the rise. He had made a name in town and in the party with his partnership's newspaper, the *Shield and Banner*, a stridently pro-Democrat newspaper.[28] He held elected posts in society, including President of The Richland County Mechanics Society in 1841[29] and an Adjutant (equivalent of Lieutenant) in the Ohio militia artillery based in Mansfield in June 1842.[30] He was called to speak on the stump for candidates, which was the usual manner of campaigning in the mid-19th century.[31] While on the stump and studying law, A. S. Maxwell crossed paths and became an acquaintance of Samuel Jordan Kirkwood, who was apparently of a similar mind. Archibald's popularity grew. He was asked on several occasions to run on the Democratic ticket in the late 1840s and early 1850s. But Archibald turned down such opportunities to run for public office on the Democratic Party ticket, because he did not support the party platform that permitted expansion of slavery into the Western Territories.[32] He eventually left the Democratic Party over this issue at the start of the Civil War.

In 1842, misfortune dashed his hopes and dreams, altering perhaps forever the course of his life. He fell ill with what he claimed was laryngitis.[33] The illness "destroyed his voice and resulted in his having to leave his collegiate course and abandon his favorite profession, the law." Many years later, he would describe it to his biographers that he abandoned the law with "with deep regrets, almost remorse." [34] Having been forced by circumstances to give up the law, he would instead become a doctor and surgeon.

After recovering from this sickness, Archibald continued to suffer recurring periods of illness. Later in his life, he refused a commission as an assistant surgeon in the 1848 War with Mexico on account of "poor health."[35] When he left Ohio in 1852, he claimed "his health [was] failing." In June 1862 during the Civil War, he returned to Davenport from the hospitals in Tennessee and Mississippi with "his health being much impaired."[36] It is possible that he suffered from a chronic illness that grew worse at times of high stress but was never diagnosed.

Whether he suffered from a chronic illness is unknown. It is also possible that he drove himself sick with his relentless work ethic. Dr. Cantwell, a former apprentice of his, wrote of him in memoriam, "It was a wonder to me how he endured the fatigue he was called upon to pass through; he would never refuse a call if possibly able to go, and it seemed to me that he went at night as much as in the day. At times he would seem completely worn out; would think he would not be able to be out for days; then, after a few hours of sleep, he would be up and visiting patients who were not half so sick as himself."[37]

The illness in 1842 at the age of 24 caused him to move back to Berlin, Ohio, to his family, after more than five years away. There, he chose to pursue a career in medicine. The move and the change of professional focus caused Archibald much distress. Over 30 years later, Archibald would recall that he pursued a career in medicine with a local doctor, John M. Cook, M.D., in Berlin, Ohio, "with many misgivings." [38]

Misgivings or not, he pursued his career in medicine with the same passion for education and training that he had shown with his other professions. At the time, two years of medical college plus training with a practicing doctor (preceptor) was considered the new and emerging standard.[39] He met this standard when he graduated from the Western Reserve College in Hudson, Ohio, in 1848.[40] By that time, he also completed a five-year apprenticeship with his preceptor, John Cook.

After graduation, he joined with his preceptor in opening a practice in Berlin, Ohio. Because he had married John Cook's stepdaughter, Charlotte Hough, in 1847, he joined the family business. In keeping with that tradition, he would later make his younger brother, Dr. David Maxwell, a partner in the business in 1850. The practice of medicine in rural Berlin, Ohio, was grueling and required him to take "long rides day and night." [41] Despite the hectic schedule and work conditions, he and his wife had three children born while they lived in Berlin.

In 1852, Archibald decided that he was interested in striking out to the frontier, but he wanted to travel a bit before settling on a new place. By this point in his career, he had gained a sufficiently prominent reputation that people in need of his medical opinion and surgical services would call him to visit and perform surgeries for sick residents in Indiana and Western Ohio towns. Building on this already far-distant business, he travelled for several years to western and southwestern states (likely Indiana, Illinois, Iowa, and Missouri) "performing many of the finer operations of surgery" and scouting for a new place to live.

After his search, he chose the growing and expanding city of Davenport, Iowa. He and his family relocated there on April 3, 1855, likely because the property boom provided the illusion of an opportunity to make money on real estate investments.[42] During the period of his search from 1852–1854, Davenport was particularly attractive, as the population of the town grew from 3,500 in 1852 to 6,000 in 1854.[43] The growth, with the resulting demand for increased housing, drove the price of land higher. Before moving to Iowa, Archibald liquidated his property in Berlin, Ohio, and invested "considerable money in real estate at a time when everything was high."[44] He also must have borrowed a considerable sum for real estate and improvements. In 1855–56, he spent "most of his time and means in improvements" of his buildings and his city lots as well as his real estate outside the city. [45]

When all seemed settled for Archibald in his new home, disaster struck. The financial crisis in 1857 caused a massive liquidity crisis in the United States and United Kingdom.[46] Many U.S. banks failed, and others stopped lending money for speculative land investments in the West. As it did many others, the financial crisis hit Archibald hard. To pay his debts, he sold "the greater part of his considerable real estate to meet his obligations, [but] every cent was paid."[47] In fact, this process would take several years. In 1862, while he was serving his country in the Civil War, his creditors seized and sold his land to pay his debts.[48]

After he moved to Davenport in 1855, he initially chose to practice less medicine and invest more in real estate. He originally intended to set up a medical practice specializing in specific surgeries.[49] He ran an advertisement "A.S. Maxwell, M.D. Surgeon, Oculist & Operator Tenotomy & Plastic Surgery" with references in the *Davenport Daily Gazette* starting in 1855. According to the newspaper, he performed operations for the removal of cataracts; ptosis (drooping eyelids); strabismus (misalignment of the eye) or squintings; hare lip; club foot; contracted limbs etc.[50] However, his financial reverses in 1857 required him to abandon his specialized practice, and change back to the general practice model that he had used before he left Berlin, Ohio.[51]

He quickly became established in the physician community in Davenport as a doctor and surgeon of experience and good reputation. He was a founding member of the Scott County Medical Society in October 1858.[52] He also was part of a team of doctors that successfully performed the first tracheotomy in Davenport in 1859.[53] In March–April 1860, he was part of surgical teams that performed two reported amputations to remove timorous growths and diseased bone.[54] In October 1860, he joined his general medical practice with Dr. Tomson.[55]

In Davenport, he also demonstrated a continued commitment to public education and became a leader in the community on this issue. From 1859 to 1860, he was elected to the "Board of Presidents of Township Districts of Scott County" for Davenport City Township.[56] The Board governed the common schools of Scott County, which were attended by 1,000 children in the 1859–60 school year. He served first as Board Secretary and rose to Chairman in the fall of 1859, just as controversy and crisis struck the Scott County public school system, threatening the closure of the schools.

By September 1859, the Scott County public schools were out of money for "fuel or other contingencies" and faced a "total stoppage of all [county] public schools." A school tax levy was proposed to close the funding gap. A "very warm" controversy arose at the September 24th meeting, and the tax levy was defeated.[57] In a Board meeting following the defeat, Archibald, as Chairman, led the board to try again on October 8th. The October 8th public meeting was widely attended, and the tax levy to pay for the remainder of the 1859–60 school year passed by a wide margin.[58]

Archibald's devotion and leadership in the public sphere as shown by his stint on the school board, and his expertise as a surgeon would be needed to answer the call for medical and sanitary needs of Union soldiers, and in particular, the Iowa soldiers. His prior public service on the school board positioned him to be entrusted by his fellow Davenport citizens on two separate expeditions to the front to help find their wounded and send them home. He along with others—most prominently his fellow Iowa state sanitary agent, Annie Turner Wittenmyer— answered the call to give aid to the fathers, sons, friends, and neighbors who had volunteered to fight and preserve the union. Archibald faced rebel bullets, and camp diseases. He also witnessed the dangers created by the Union Army's utter failure to plan, prepare, and provide even the basic level of medical care possible in the 1860s for its wounded and sick soldiers in the early years of the American Civil War in the Western Theater.

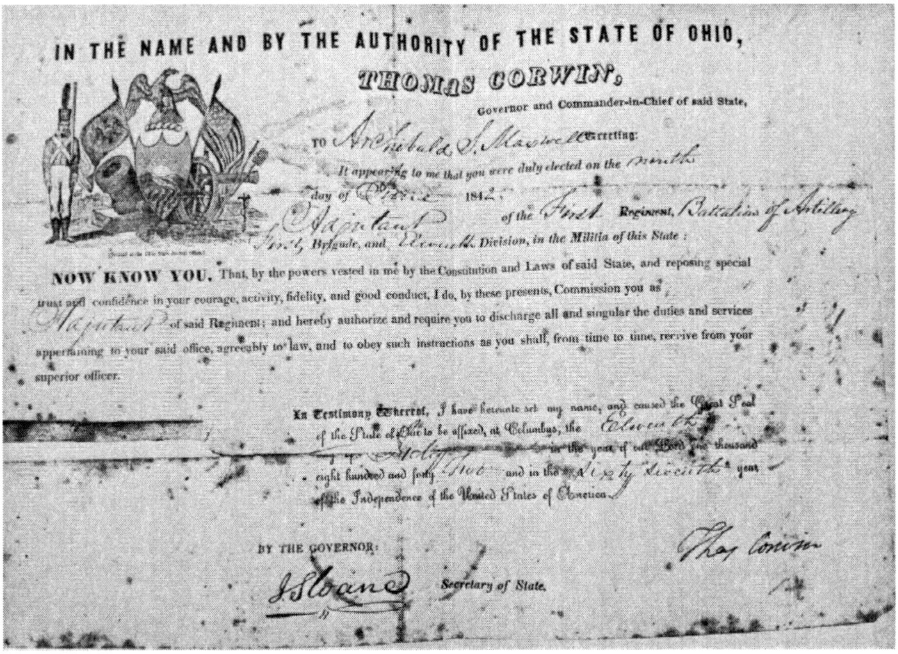
IN THE NAME AND BY THE AUTHORITY OF THE STATE OF OHIO,

THOMAS CORWIN,

Governor and Commander-in-Chief of said State,

TO Archibald S. Maxwell Greeting:

It appearing to me that you were duly elected on the ninth day of [illegible] 1842, Adjutant of the First Regiment, Battalion of Artillery First Brigade, and Eleventh Division, in the Militia of this State:

NOW KNOW YOU, That, by the powers vested in me by the Constitution and Laws of said State, and reposing special trust and confidence in your courage, activity, fidelity, and good conduct, I do, by these presents, Commission you as Adjutant of said Regiment; and hereby authorize and require you to discharge all and singular the duties and services appertaining to your said office, agreeably to law, and to obey such instructions as you shall, from time to time, receive from your superior officer.

In Testimony Whereof, I have hereunto set my name, and caused the Great Seal of the State of Ohio to be affixed, at Columbus, the Eleventh day of [illegible] in the year of our Lord one thousand eight hundred and forty Two and in the Sixty Seventh year of the Independence of the United States of America.

BY THE GOVERNOR:

Thos Corwin

J Sloane Secretary of State.

Ohio State Militia Certificate given to Archibald S. Maxwell on his election as Adjutant in 1842.

CHAPTER 2:
The Tragedies of Early 1861

The year 1861 began in tragedy for Archibald and the United States. The United States that he loved began to fall apart after the election of Abraham Lincoln in November 1860. South Carolina left the Union in December. In January 1861, the states of Mississippi, Alabama, Georgia, and Louisiana followed. Texas seceded on February 1st. The drumbeat of war began to sound.

Meanwhile, personal tragedy struck. In January 1861, Archibald's sister Margaret was found to have very advanced breast cancer.[59] She was 57 years old. Archibald returned to Berlin, Ohio, to try to save her.

Margaret was important to Archibald. She was the adult sister who had helped their mother with her eight minor children, including four-year-old Archibald, when their father John died. Archibald grew up in Berlin, Ohio, near his sister. He established his first medical practice in Berlin, Ohio, as well, and began his family there before he moved to Davenport, Iowa. A daughter of his, Elta Margaret Maxwell, carried her middle name.

As reported in her March 21, 1861, obituary in the Holmes County Republican, the cancerous lump in Margaret's right breast had been discovered 2 years before, probably by her and Archibald's younger brother Dr. David Maxwell. At the time, the growth had been characterized as "gradual...but not exciting any decidedly serious apprehensions." By January 1861, the cancer had advanced and her health began to fail. "Medical treatment was instituted," probably by her brother David, "but little check however was made upon [the cancer]'s depressing influence on her system." David or another family member summoned Archibald from faraway Davenport, Iowa. A "council of a number physicians," which likely included Archibald, David, and their mentor Dr. Cook (Archibald's father-in-law), came together and recommended a mastectomy, or as it was written in 1861, amputation of "the mammillary gland." On February 16, 1861, Archibald performed the surgery, which was deemed successful. For a few days, Margaret began to show "marked symptoms of a speedy recovery," and then infection set in. The infection "baffled the untiring energies and skill of the attending physicians [likely Archibald and David] as well as the most potent remedies." The language hints at the Herculean efforts of the brother doctors trying to keep a much beloved elder sister on this side of the veil. [60] Unfortunately, ten days after the surgery, on February 26, 1861, Margaret slipped away.

As Archibald operated to try to save his sister, politicians in the South moved to solidify the dismemberment of the United States. Jefferson Davis of Mississippi was inaugurated as President of the fledging Confederate States of America on February 18, 1861.

On April 12, 1861, Confederate troops began the bombardment of Fort Sumter in Charleston Harbor. On April 14, 1861, Fort Sumter surrendered, and President Lincoln called for 75,000 volunteers to suppress the rebellion. Shortly thereafter, Virginia, North Carolina, Tennessee, and Arkansas joined the Confederate States of America. President Lincoln increased his call for volunteers, and the states raised more volunteer regiments to combat the expanding rebellion.

As the secession crisis deepened, Archibald's family suffered two additional personal tragedies. On April 20, 1861, Elta Margaret, aged 1 year and 28 days, caught pneumonia and followed her Aunt Margaret into the next world.[61] Archibald's father-in-law, Dr. John M. Cook, died of bronchitis at age 54 in Berlin, Ohio, in the same month.[62] Dr. John M. Cook was more than just Archibald's father-in-law and stepfather of his wife, Charlotte. Dr. Cook had taken in and trained a young Archibald as a doctor after Archibald could no longer pursue his chosen profession in the law due to illness. Dr. Cook had also trained Archibald's younger brother David to be a doctor. Dr. Cook had made Archibald a partner in his medical partnership after Archibald had married his stepdaughter and finished medical college.

Shortly after Dr. Cook's death, the war became personal for Archibald and his wife, Charlotte. His wife's half-brother, John F. Cook, left medical school and answered President Lincoln's second call for volunteers on May 3, 1861. [63] He enlisted in the 19th Ohio volunteer regiment as a private, even though he had not yet completed the settling of his father's estate. With his brother-in-law's enlistment, Archibald and his wife had a personal reason to be worried when news of major engagements involving Ohio Volunteer Regiments trickled in. The war that Archibald's brother-in-law volunteered to join was still new.

The American Civil War turned out to be vastly different from the prior wars fought in North America. The two sides engaged in massive mobilizations of their populations for near-total war. Organized and systemized efforts at home to support troops were designed to maximize the number of troops deployed on the frontline and to sustain their deployment for significant periods of time. Archibald's efforts on behalf of the Union cause as a doctor and a surgeon and his participant in various sanitary organizations were aspects of this.

Also, telegraphs, railroads, and steam-powered ships improved communication and movement of information, armies, and supplies. News of a battle arrived over the telegraph, and within days of the battle, people in places like Davenport arranged to send and deliver relief to help with the sick and wounded.[64] The increased speed of communication and transport made it easier to move and concentrate large bodies of troops over long distances.

However, few people, including army officers, understood the effects of the increased speed of communication (telegraph) and transportation (railroad and steamship) at the beginning of the war. Faster communication and transportation enabled larger armies to concentrate to fight bigger battles, with the potential for higher casualties. For instance, the army failed to appreciate that armies of a larger size could not live off the land as effectively as smaller armies had by foraging for the fruits and vegetables to keep them healthy.[65] Also, larger armies were larger petri dishes for diseases, when they did not maintain good sanitary practices, which was the case with the army, particularly early in the war.[66]

At the beginning of the war, the Army Medical Corps led by the octogenarian surgeon general, a veteran of the war of 1812, was not ready and capable to supply the kind of treatment in the field that was possible and expected by people.[67] This contributed to rise to local, state, regional, and national sanitary commissions to fill in the gap.

However, at the time Archibald's brother-in-law, John Cook, volunteered in May 1861, many on both sides still believed the war would be short, which made the need for medical assistance appear less immediate. In the beginning, people treated the war like a spectator sport, riding out to watch at the Battle of Bull Run, and watching the bombardment of Fort Sumter. Also, the Union volunteers had not been in the field long enough for word of the medical care deficiencies and the general unhealthy nature of their camps to come back to the home front.

Toward the end of 1861, the *Daily Davenport Gazette* in Archibald's hometown of Davenport printed letters from the soldiers at the front, reporting outbreaks of diseases like measles and the terrible condition of the hospitals and medical aid.[68] These articles, along with stump speeches by activists in the sanitation movement, like Annie Wittenmyer and Reverend Kynett, began to generate interest by Archibald and others to do something about the deplorable medical conditions and the lack of care provided by the Army Medical Corps.[69]

CHAPTER 3:
An Iowa Rivalry—The Competing Organizations for Soldiers' Relief

It appears Archibald did not get involved with sanitary commissions and soldiers' relief organizations until local, male citizens began to form a soldiers' relief organization in his home town of Davenport in February 1862. It was eventually called the Scott County Soldiers' Relief Association. The Scott County Soldiers Relief Association would be one of many such local organizations which included ladies aid societies (mainly women members) and soldiers' relief organizations (mainly male members). These organizations were formed at the local level to gather donations of needed medical assistance goods, raise cash donations, and also identify willing, capable volunteers to provide medical services at hospitals. These local organizations then funneled their donations to a state organization, which in turn sent them on to a sanitary commission of regional or national scope.

In mid-1861, Archibald returned to Davenport from Ohio after burying his relatives. He resumed his Davenport medical practice, and continued to advertise his practice in the *Davenport Daily Gazette*. He participated in the Scott County Medical Society and on the local Board of Education's Examining Committee for the 1861 school year.[70] He had volunteered for both organizations before the beginning of the Civil War. Basically, the rising tide of war had yet to change the normal patterns of Archibald's life. Archibald was not terribly different than many other people who remained on the home front in late 1861.

Although Archibald resumed his usual pattern of life in 1861, people like Annie Wittenmyer in the soldiers' aid movement made significant strides organizationally. In that year, important medical assistance organizations, called sanitary commissions, formed at the national, regional, state, and local level. These organizations had a significant influence on Archibald when he finally did begin to participate in the movement in 1862. At the state level, Archibald would play an important role in the rivalry, competition, and intrigue between Reverend A. J.

Kynett's organization and Annie Wittenmyer's organization. At a regional and national level, Archibald had at least a passing acquaintance with the three main organizations: the U.S. Sanitary Commission, Western Sanitary Commission, and the Christian Commission. The *Iowa Journal of History and Politics* article "Relief Work During Civil War" by Earl S. Fulbrook in the April 1918 Volume 16 No. 2 provides a excellent summary of the various organizations, but plays down the rivalry that existed between them. Also, the U.S. Sanitary Commission, the U.S. Sanitary Commission in the Valley of the Mississippi, and the Western Sanitary Commission all published extensive histories of their work shortly after the war.

Nationally, the U.S. Sanitary Commission formed in April–May 1861 in New York City. The U.S. Sanitary Commission was the largest of the commissions, and it sought to remedy the deficiencies in the army and the Army Medical Corps at the beginning of the war. After some wrangling, the organizers convinced the Department of War to issue an order in June 1861 that gave them the authority to provide sanitary relief and medical assistance to the Union volunteers but not the regular army.[71]

Regionally, the rise of the Western Sanitary Commission in St. Louis, Missouri, in September 1861 was important to Archibald and Annie Wittenmyer, with whom he worked later in the war. As noted earlier, the Western Sanitary Commission arose in St. Louis after the people saw the depth of the army's lack of preparedness following the Battle of Wilson's Creek and other engagements in Missouri. Major General John Fremont, then the senior army officer in the theater, appointed the Western Sanitary Commissioners and set out the scope of their assistance. At the time of the Western Sanitary Commission's creation, the U.S. Sanitary Commission was absent from the scene, giving the sense that the West had been left to make up for the Army Medical Corps' failings on its own.

The competition and rivalry between the Western and the U.S. Sanitary Commissions began in the fall of 1861. In late September 1861, the U.S. Sanitary Commission finally managed to send its agent, Dr. Newberry, west of the Appalachian Mountains. Shortly after arriving in the West, Dr. Newberry traveled to St. Louis to "offer" the Western Sanitary Commission to join the U.S. Sanitary Commission under his management. The Western Sanitary Commission declined to join with the U.S. Sanitary Commission.[72] The two organizations eventually agreed that the Western Sanitary Commission would address sanitary efforts from the Mississippi River west, and the U.S. Sanitary Commission would address sanitary issues east of the Mississippi River. [73]

The competition between the Western Sanitary Commission and the U.S. Sanitary Commission for donations and distribution of goods through their supply systems played a role in the politics of the two Iowa state organizations from 1861–1863. The Keokuk Ladies Aid Society network, led by Mrs. Annie Wittenmyer, was the first Iowa organization, and it sent its donations mainly through the Western Sanitary Commission in St. Louis. [74] The second organization, the Iowa Army State Sanitary Commission, led by Reverend A. J. Kynett, sent its donations mainly through the U.S. Sanitary Commission.[75] Archibald became intimately familiar with these rivalries. He worked with both Reverend Kynett and Annie Wittenmyer. He later assisted Annie Wittenmyer in her efforts to disrupt Reverend Kynett's attempts to, as Annie Wittenmyer put it in her letter, "embarrass" her and the sanitary affairs movement in Iowa.[76]

The Keokuk Ladies Aid Society's network of ladies aid societies arose organically as a grassroots movement due to Annie Wittenmyer's leadership and the efforts of the Keokuk Ladies Aid Society to establish a statewide network to gather and distribute needed sanitary goods to Iowa troops. A January 1862 report by the Iowa Army State Sanitary Commission described the Keokuk network as consisting of ladies aid societies at Keokuk, Burlington, Davenport, and Dubuque, as well as unnamed ladies aid societies in the interior that sent contributions through the Keokuk Ladies Aid Society, including the ladies aid society in Iowa City.[77] Basically, the ladies aid societies in these cities represented organizations from major population centers. In January 1862, this network funneled its donations to the Western Sanitary Commission in St. Louis.[78]

Annie Wittenmyer and the Keokuk Ladies Aid Society preceded the creation of Iowa Army State Sanitary Commission. Annie Wittenmyer and the Keokuk Ladies Aid Society began to provide sanitary aid in the summer of 1861. The City of Keokuk's location at the junction of the Mississippi and Des Moines Rivers likely assisted the Keokuk Ladies Aid Society in building its network. Keokuk was an important node for logistics and communication, particularly in the early part of the war, as many Iowa volunteer regiments gathered there before leaving Iowa for the war in Missouri. Moreover, Annie Wittenmyer began to reach out to other ladies aid societies around the state to coordinate their efforts. She followed the Iowa 2nd Regiment down into Missouri in August 1861 and learned of the regiment's needs. In September 1861, she went out again for ten days with needed medical supplies for the Iowa regiments, returned to gather more supplies, and left again for three weeks.[79] Also, in September 1861, the Keokuk Ladies Aid Society published a circular asking ladies aid societies in the state of Iowa to unite to send supplies for soldiers' relief.[80]

Annie Wittenmyer and her network were particularly adept at learning what the soldiers needed, telling the people back home, and then personally delivering the aid. Soldiers, surgeons, and officers sang her praises in letters published in newspapers at home. Archibald valued her organization's aid when he was a surgeon and followed her lead in delivering goods when acting as a sanitary agent. Part of Annie Wittenmyer's political power arose from her ability to deliver supplies and make that connection to home personally, or through the management of others like Archibald.

The second organization, the Iowa Army State Sanitary Commission, which was also called the Iowa State Sanitary Commission, was led by Reverend A. J. Kynett as Corresponding Secretary. Samuel J. Kirkwood, governor of Iowa, appointed the commission in October 1861. It represented an attempt to manage the sanitary affairs movement from the top down. The Iowa Army State Sanitary Commission sent nearly all of its aid to the U.S. Sanitary Commission's regional office in Chicago, Illinois.[81]

Governor Kirkwood, for reasons not known today, determined that a state commission was necessary, despite the efforts of the network led by the Keokuk Ladies Aid Society. Governor Kirkwood sent a letter to Reverend A. J. Kynett, dated October 10, 1861. In that missive, Governor Kirkwood observed that "voluntary associations are being organized with a view to provide our sick and wounded soldiers with articles essential to their comfort and not furnished by the government." He likely meant organizations like the Keokuk Ladies Aid Society and its network. He asked Reverend A. J. Kynett "to encourage the formation of such societies ... in the various communities in the state and perfect a system by which contributions thus made will reach those of our citizen soldiers who may be in need."[82] Governor Kirkwood expressed a desire that "societies already formed and hereafter organized" to cooperate with Reverend Kynett in accomplishing this task. Accordingly, he expected the state commission to act as a central coordinating point for all the local aid societies like the Keokuk Ladies Aid Society. Governor Kirkwood was trying to pull apart the informal network created by the Keokuk Ladies Aid Society.

Reverend Kynett responded to the governor shortly thereafter with a letter "recommending that a State Sanitary Commission be constituted" similar to the U.S. Sanitary Commission "with a view of making it ultimately auxiliary" to the U.S. Sanitary Commission. In the letter to Governor Kirkwood, Reverend A. J. Kynett proposed 13 men from around Iowa as part of the commission, including Prof. J. C. Hughes, M.D. as president and himself as the corresponding secretary. On October

13, 1861, the governor appointed the proposed Army Sanitary Commission for the state of Iowa from Reverend A. J. Kynett's slate of names.[83] Reverend A. J. Kynett took a position parallel to Annie Wittenmyer's. Reverend Kynett's list did not include Annie Wittenmyer or anyone from her organization. It has been suggested that Annie Wittenmyer was not considered for the Commission because she was a woman, and in Victorian society, such a position was not deemed proper.[84] Annie Wittenmyer and her organization would challenge that notion.

On October 28, 1861, the governor, on behalf of the Iowa State Army Sanitary Commission, published an article in newspapers throughout the state that explained the Iowa State Sanitary Commission's purpose.[85] The commission duplicated the efforts of Annie Wittenmyer's organization. Moreover, the Iowa State Army Sanitary Commission intended to shift donations away from the Western Sanitary Commission in St. Louis, where many Iowa regiments were stationed, in favor of the U.S. Sanitary Commission.

Annie Wittenmyer's organization—the Keokuk Ladies Aid Society and its affiliate branches—struck back in an unsigned *The Weekly Gate City* article published in November 1861. The article lambasted the Iowa State Sanitary Commission and explained that the Keokuk Ladies Aid Society already had been doing the work the Commission sought to do and had been quite successful at it, making the Commission duplicative and unnecessary.[86]

Even if the Commission was duplicative, there was enough work for everyone. The medical news from the troops in the field was terrible. Volunteer regiments suffered from outbreaks of measles and other infectious diseases. Hospitals in Missouri at first were not well supplied until donations came in to alleviate the matter.[87] In its January 1862 report of conditions in the field, the Commission concluded that "the hospitals are far from being supplied with necessary articles." They predicted that the medical supply shortage would only get worse with "every engagement and every march that is at all severe and long."[88]

Reverend Kynett returned from the field, published the report, and began to give lectures on the benefit of soldiers' aid societies. For instance, he gave a lecture on January 21, 1862, at the Metropolitan Hall in Davenport for the benefit of the ladies soldiers' aid society. He spoke of the conditions of Iowa soldiers in different hospitals to raise awareness of the troops' needs.

Despite his efforts, Reverend Kynett had limited success in uniting the soldiers' aid groups around the state of Iowa. The list at the end of the Commission's

January 1862 report contained the names of 72 organizations, but they were all from the interior part of the state, which had lower population. None of the larger, wealthier Mississippi River towns of Keokuk, Burlington, Muscatine, Davenport, Clinton, or Dubuque were on his list. Most of the groups came from small, rural villages that remain so to this day, including the author's hometown of Central City. Reverend Kynett's frustration led him to embark on efforts to undermine the Keokuk Ladies Aid Society and provide political legitimacy for the Iowa State Sanitary Commission.

CHAPTER 4:
Off to Rescue the Wounded From Fort Donelson

Archibald entered into this unsettled rivalry when he attended another public Davenport Citizen's Meeting at Le Claire House on February 19, 1862, "for the purpose of devising ways and means for relief of the wounded at the taking of Fort Donelson." The Citizen's Meeting was called because a telegraph had arrived with the word that local Iowa boys in the Iowa 2nd Infantry had made a heroic charge and paid the price. Now they needed and had asked for help. Davenport prepared to send a Relief Committee.

Nearly two weeks before the February 19th Davenport meeting that Archibald attended, General Grant began his offensive campaign against Confederate Fort Heiman, Fort Henry on the Tennessee River, and Fort Donelson on the Cumberland River. [89] Confederates under General Albert Sidney Johnston constructed these forts as part of a defensive line to prevent the Union from using its gunboats to invade the South.

On February 5th–6th 1862, General Grant captured Fort Heiman and Fort Henry with few casualties. He then quickly moved to capture Fort Donelson only 11 miles from Fort Henry. The capture of Fort Donelson proved more difficult. General Grant succeeded in capturing it on February 16th after a fight spread out over three days.

The capture of those three forts broke the Confederate defensive line. It opened up the Tennessee River and Cumberland River, allowing the Union to threaten Nashville and penetrate into Mississippi and Alabama by river. It made it possible to cut a key east–west, Memphis and Charleston Railroad where the railroad crossed the rivers.[90]

In the Battle of Fort Donelson, the Union suffered over 2,000 wounded and 500 dead. Some of these causalities came from General McClernand's attempt to capture a battery, which resulted in great loss on February 13th. The balance was largely suffered during the battle on February 15th, when the Confederates attempted to break out of the fort.

On February 15th, the Iowa Second Infantry Regiment was part of Grant's army that had the Confederates penned in at Fort Donelson. At 2:00 p.m. on that day, Colonel Tuttle received an order "to storm the fortifications" of Fort Donelson, according to his regimental report. [91] He ordered his regiment to fix bayonets and advance across the ground to the outer fortification ring of earthen walls. The regiment's 630 soldiers steadily advanced up the hill in an "unbroken line" across the ground into heavy Confederate fire from Fort Donelson. [92] Soon after the advance began, Confederates singled out the men bearing the regimental flags leading the charge. They shot Color Sergeant H. B. Doolittle multiple times. He fell gravely wounded. Others who bore the colors before them were also shot. Despite the losses, the Iowa 2nd covered the ground and scaled the earthen walls of the outer breastworks. When they reached the top, the Confederates broke, "flying before [them] except a few who were promptly put to the bayonet." The regiment fired into the retreating Confederates and charged the Confederate encampment. Other regiments followed up to consolidate the breach. For the privilege of having been the first to breach Fort Donelson's outer defensive works, the Iowa 2nd paid in blood, suffering 40 dead and 160 wounded. In addition to the Iowa 2nd, other Iowa regiments—the 7th and 14th—were engaged in the fight.

With the fort breached and the Confederate breakout attempt contained, the Confederate General Simon Bolivar Buckner reluctantly accepted General Grant's terms to unconditionally surrender Fort Donelson on February 16, 1862.

After the battle, the citizens of Davenport received a telegram requesting aid for the Iowa wounded.[93] The request to send aid led to the February 19th meeting at the Le Claire House in Davenport, three days after the surrender.

At the Le Claire House meeting, the male citizens of Davenport devised ways to provide relief to the wounded and sick at Fort Donelson and selected local people to provide that assistance.[94] Archibald attended the meeting, as did many other men in Davenport. He may have attended because the Governor asked him to attend and volunteer. Archibald may also have attended and volunteered to help because he was a strong supporter of the Union and had long-held, deep-seated beliefs that slavery was wrong.

The Relief Committee was keen to see that the wounded from Companies B and C of the Iowa 2nd Infantry Regiment received attention. The citizens at first did not consider sending surgeons to provide medical relief until it was suggested by someone that it might be wise. The citizens added Archibald and Dr. Stephenson to the Davenport Relief Committee. After some thought, Dr. Stephenson was replaced by Dr. McCarn, because a doctor of German ancestry was deemed a more appropriate choice given the high number German-Americans enlisted in Companies B and C.

At the meeting, the Davenport Relief Committee was instructed to telegraph from Cairo, Illinois, with the names of the killed and wounded. As the Committee prepared to leave Davenport, a telegram was sent ahead to the Iowa 2nd Infantry Regiment to inform them that help was on the way.

On February 20th, less than a day after the Wednesday, the appointed Davenport Relief Committee, consisting of Mr. Willard Barrows, Mr. L. J. Center, Judge Linderman, Colonel Ira Gifford, Mr. L. C. Burwell, Dr. Archibald Maxwell, and Dr. McCarn, journeyed out by steamer down the Mississippi to Cairo, Illinois. They carried with them medical supplies and money. The account of much of their trip appeared as a report by Mr. L. C. Burwell in the *Davenport Daily Gazette* on March 8, 1862, and a report by Dr. Maxwell in the *Davenport Daily Gazette* on March 22, 1862.

The Davenport Relief Committee arrived at Cairo, Illinois—the strategic city at the junction of the Ohio and Mississippi Rivers—at 7:00 p.m. on Friday, February 22, 1862. They sought and found an Iowa regimental surgeon that they knew in Cairo, and he let them sleep in the Cairo Hospital that night. Less than one week had passed since the surrender of Fort Donelson.

Before they went to bed on Friday, they earnestly sought information on casualties in the Iowa 2nd Infantry, particularly news of Companies B and C, which were from Davenport. The group relied on sources of information about causalities that were, at best, unofficial, although it may have been the only information available at the time. They interviewed the Quartermaster, who was from Iowa, and his aide, Mr. Morrison, for information, and telegraphed that as a part of their first report back to Davenport. Later, the group sent a second telegraph passing along information gleaned from one of the Iowa wounded that arrived in Cairo on a boat.

Relief committees like the one from Davenport and their supplies were needed at Fort Donelson because the army came up short in planning for its wounded and sick. From the remarks in General Grant's memoirs and the accounts of the U.S. Sanitary Commission in the Valley of the Mississippi, it is evident that logistical planning and making provisions for adequate hospital tents and other supplies was not a priority yet. General Grant remarked after the beginning of the battle for Fort Donelson, "Up to this time the surgeons with the army had no difficulty in finding room in houses near our line for the sick and wounded; but now [after McClernand's assault] hospitals were overcrowded."[95] General Grant's comment that the field hospital ran out of space when the fighting started makes evident that the army and its Medical Corps had not seriously planned post-battle medical treatment.

General Grant in his memoirs attempts to defend the level of care provided by stating that due to the surgeons, the "suffering was not so great as it might have been."[96] Grant's compliment is likely attributable to Medical Director Hewitt's more efficient and organized approach to dressing the wounded and moving them back to one of four field hospitals for treatment. This new centralized process turned out to be better than having the wounded treated in the more dispersed regimental hospitals.[97] Nevertheless, General Grant's comment admits there was great suffering. It is not much of a compliment to indicate that it might have been worse.

While the triage during the battle may have been better, the sustained care of the wounded after the victory was not. When the U.S. Sanitary Commission group from Cincinnati arrived at the Fort Donelson battlefield four days after the battle, they described the condition of the wounded as "deplorable" with some having "undressed wounds," a lack of bandages or extra clothing, insufficient medicine, and insufficient hospital food, and overworked surgeons.[98]

The wounded in the Fort Donelson battle spent four or five days in these conditions before they were loaded on steamers to be transported to hospitals at Paducah, Mound City, Cairo, and St. Louis.[99] The lack of hospital space and supplies necessitated moving the wounded upriver.

Archibald and some of the Davenport Relief Committee witnessed firsthand the conditions of the wounded on these hospital boats that arrived in Cairo and Mound City. On the morning of Saturday, February 23rd, Ira Gifford, Judge Linderman, and Dr. McCarn met with Brigadier General Paine to arrange their plans to proceed further in search of Iowa wounded in need of assistance. While waiting for orders from General Paine, Archibald, Mr. L. J. Center, and Mr. Burwell boarded the steamer *Hazel Dell*, carrying 83 wounded Union soldiers from Iowa and Illinois, which had arrived in Cairo during the night. The ship had seventy sick rebel soldiers onboard as well.

The conditions on the riverboat *Hazel Dell* revealed the army's shortcomings in provisions and planning for its wounded. Archibald found "no surgeon on board in charge" of the wounded on the boat, which was strange enough that he noted it in his report. In caring for the wounded, Archibald "found our labors greatly embarrassed by the great want of all articles used for dressing wounds—lint, bandages and adhesive piaster."[100] He found many of the soldiers "whose wounds had not been dressed but once" after they were injured a week earlier. These soldiers "were mostly in the same clothes that were on them when wounded, which were stiff with blood and dust."[101] Archibald was evidently appalled by the low level of care and the failure of the army to fulfill the most basic of duties—supplying a clean change of clothes for the wounded and changing bandages regularly.

Archibald's more contemporaneous account of the terrible conditions on the river transports is similar to that provided by the U.S. Sanitary Commission in its visit to Fort Donelson. Both of these accounts contrast with those of John H. Brinton, who was the surgeon responsible in part for looking after the process of getting the wounded out of the battlefield hospital at Fort Donelson and on transports to hospitals upriver. For posterity in his memoirs written decades after the war, John Brinton claimed that the wounded were "put onboard, carefully attended to and dressed, and then moved in the hospital boats."[102] Brinton's account appears to leave important details out.

As absurd as it sounds today, the "hospital" boat probably did not have a bandage on it when it departed from the battle site at Fort Donelson to journey downriver at Cairo. According to Archibald's description in his report, the soldiers on the boat had not been bandaged during the trip, and the boat was bereft of bandages.

Archibald also noted a basic failure of the army to plan and provide meals that could be fed to the sick and wounded, or the basic utensils that might be used to feed it to them. This problem would persist for quite some time. On the *Hazel Dell* and all other boats that he checked on his trip, the army had not made any provision for the sick and wounded to "get regular *warm meals.*"[103] The army had instead provided "rations" for soldiers on the march "consisting of poor beef, ham shoulder, hard bread (with some in whole loaves), coffee, and stuff marked black tea."[104] The army had neither provided "utensils to cook with nor articles suitable to eat with." The hospital boat did not have tins, plates, knives, or spoons that could be used to feed the wounded. Thus, bereft of the proper tools and supplies, the wounded did not receive warm meals in a manner that they might best be able to eat it.

Despite these handicaps, Archibald, Mr. L. J. Center, Mr. L. C. Burwell, and some lady nurses managed to dress the 83 wounded men on the boat. The lady nurses sacrificed some of their articles of clothing for bandages. Archibald indicated that they were only able to treat the wounded because the women had divested "of such raiment and their wardrobes of all articles" to be torn up and used for bandages.[105]

After disembarking from the *Hazel Dell*, their further search for Iowa wounded required them to procure passes to travel up the Ohio River to visit hospitals at Mound City and Paducah, where they believed many of the wounded had been sent by steamer from Fort Donelson. To Mr. L. C. Burwell's surprise, the Union Army required them to enlist as volunteer surgeons and nurses before the army would issue passes for them to travel up the Ohio River. Archibald and the remainder of the party enlisted and placed themselves "exclusively under the direction of the military authorities."[106]

Despite the requirement that the group enlist, the army proved quite flexible in giving out "orders" that happened to correspond with the purpose of the group's trip. The army was desperate for medical assistance and likely willing to take whatever assistance they might get. General Paine ordered Archibald and Dr. McCarn to meet General Sherman in Paducah. The remainder of the group was ordered to Mound City Hospital to report to Surgeon Franklin.

Archibald and Dr. McCarn travelled up the Ohio River to Paducah, Kentucky, passing Mound City, Illinois. Upon their arrival at Paducah, they reported to General Sherman. They explained their mission, which did not change despite having "enlisted" in the army as volunteer surgeons. General Sherman issued Archibald and Dr. McCarn a "general permit" to visit and assist in any and all hospitals. In Paducah, Kentucky, Archibald and Dr. McCarn assisted a number of sick Iowa soldiers in the hospital who had run out of "money and means."[107]

After having assisted the sick Iowa soldiers in Paducah, Archibald was assigned to duty on a steamer moving 280 wounded from Fort Donelson to the Mound City Hospital. Upon arrival at Mound City, he was directed to report to Doctor Franklin, the surgeon in charge of Mound City Hospital.

Archibald continued to be appalled at the condition of the hospital boats transporting wounded from Fort Donelson downriver to hospitals. His report indicates conditions were similar to what he had witnessed on the *Hazel Dell* in Cairo. Many of these steamers at the time of the Battle of Fort Donelson were poorly equipped and managed. The boats had been hastily brought into service by sanitary aid commissions and state governments in response to the need.[108] He noted in his published report that the boat he was assigned to for the short trip from Paducah to Mound City "had few comforts indeed," by which he meant that the boat lacked "appropriate food, clothes, and hospital stores."[109]

Because many of the wounded had not received proper treatment since the day of the battle, they needed to have their dressings changed and emergency surgeries performed on the moving boat. Accordingly, Archibald spent the entire trip devoted to "dressing wounded, performing, and assisting to perform such operations as were urgently demanded."[110]

When the boat arrived at Mound City on Monday, February 25, 1862, the Mound City Hospital had no room for the wounded. The riverboat proceeded to Cairo for further instructions, without Archibald. He got off at Mound City as ordered, although it deprived the boat of a surgeon. In all likelihood, Archibald wanted to stay at Mound City because the remainder of the team was there. Archibald's decision to get off the boat ultimately saved the life of soldiers in the Iowa 2nd Infantry Regiment, including one who had gained notoriety in the Regiment's heroic charge on Fort Donelson.

CHAPTER 5:
Saving Color Sergeant H. B. Doolittle

When Archibald arrived at Mound City, he found the hospital in terrible condition. Color Sergeant H. B. Doolittle of the Iowa 2nd Infantry called the hospital a "living grave."[111] Archibald's assessment of the hospital is more clinical, but no less damning. Archibald noted in his report that the Mound City Hospital building "was not erected for hospital purposes; yet under the management of *experienced and trusty* Surgeons, it could be most certainly made a very great and safe retreat for the sick and wounded."[112] He regretted "exceedingly, that such cannot be now said of it."[113] As he went through the wards, he noticed that soldiers who had arrived at the hospital three or four days before were in the "same clothes they had when taken from the field."[114] Some still wore just the rags of their uniform that the surgeons had not cut away to treat their wounds.

The U.S. government had taken over existing brick warehouses in Mound City, Illinois. Surgeon John H. Brinton had been responsible for seeing that it was converted into a hospital early in the war. At the time Archibald visited it, the hospital had by his estimate 1,200 to 1,400 wounded and sick, mostly wounded. The hospital administration had divided the building into 24 wards with 50 to 80 patients per ward. By the time Archibald's report was published on March 24 in the *Davenport Daily Gazette*, the Mound City Hospital had acquired a reputation as a terrible institution. The *Davenport Daily Gazette* and other newspapers had published reports and complaints about the conditions of the Mound City Hospital from soldiers and visitors. Archibald considered those reports to be generally accurate with what he had witnessed moving through the wards. Archibald's assessment of the Mound City Hospital and conditions in Cairo echoed other surgeons' views, including Surgeon John H. Brinton, who had established the hospital at Mound City.[115]

Shortly after arrival at Mound City, Archibald reported to Dr. Franklin, who assigned him "hospital duties agreeable to the tenor of General Sherman's permit."[116] At the hospital, Archibald found his "time almost taken up with attentions to Iowa soldiers."[117] While it seems unusual that Archibald focused on Iowa wounded to the exclusion of others, it was quite a common practice.

In the erysipelas ward, Archibald stumbled across Color Sergeant Harry B. Doolittle, who had been wounded carrying the flag in the 2nd Infantry Regiment's charge to take Fort Donelson. He had been shot in three places (lower abdomen, left shoulder, and calf of his leg).[118] He was apparently doing well, considering the circumstances, until he developed erysipelas, probably related to skin infections at the site of the gunshot wounds. Erysipelas is an acute infection with skin rash, known today to be caused by bacteria, that can cause high fevers, shaking, chills, fatigue, headaches, and vomiting. Dr. Franklin's team had him moved to a ward of 50 to 80 other wounded suffering from a similar infection. According to H. B. Doolittle, Dr. Franklin and staff told him that he had twelve hours to live.[119]

Archibald did not approve of the manner in which Dr. Franklin and his staff were treating H. B. Doolittle. According to Mr. L. C. Burwell, Archibald found the ward to be "a very unfavorable place for him."[120] Mr. L. C. Burwell left the impression that Archibald did not think H. B. Doolittle's chance of recovery was good in the hospital. In his later report, Archibald did not provide much more detail other than to say that he had found H. B. Doolittle in the erysipelas ward "in a most precarious condition" and had "recommended his removal to better quarters." In all likelihood, Archibald confronted Dr. Franklin and his staff and got permission to move the color sergeant out of the hospital for treatment.

The Davenport Relief Committee obtained a private room for H. B. Doolittle in the house of Mrs. Magill in Mound City. According to Mr. L. C. Burwell's report, H. B. Doolittle proceeded to "improve immediately" upon moving to the private room. The Relief Committee likely viewed the change of location to be the reason for his improvement. While the mere changing of location to the private room might be unlikely to explain his improvement, it is more likely that he received better care in the private room. The people in the room caring for him may have provided more fluids and better food than he received in the ward.

When Archibald and others of the Davenport Relief Committee left Mound City on other duties, Judge Linderman and Mr. L. J. Center remained to nurse him back to health. Color Sergeant H. B. Doolittle survived his wounds.[121] He eventually became Captain in the Iowa 20th Infantry and survived the war to die in 1896. After recovering at Mrs. Magill's house, he was moved to a hospital in Cincinnati. His letter to the *Davenport Democrat and News* published on March 22nd credited his survival to the intervention and care of the Davenport Relief Committee, which included Archibald.[122]

The treatment of Color Sergeant Harry B. Doolittle became a prime example of the Davenport Relief Committee's dissatisfaction with the medical care at the Mound City Hospital. Shortly after the Relief Committee left, the complaints about Mound City Hospital and Dr. Franklin's management, or rather lack of management, grew.

CHAPTER 6: Journeying Up the Ohio River with Wounded from the Iowa 2ND

Even though the Relief Committee had saved H. B. Doolittle and others at Mound City, they had not fully accomplished the task entrusted to them by their fellow citizens in Davenport; other Iowa wounded needed their help. Many more Iowa wounded remained to be located in order to inform their families of their whereabouts. Having seen to the worst of the wounded in Mound City, the Davenport Relief Committee split up to cover more ground on Tuesday, February 26, 1862. Ira Gifford and Dr. McCarn proceeded down the Cumberland River to Fort Donelson, where they met up with Iowa Governor Kirkwood and other Iowa state officials visiting the Iowa regiments.[123]

In addition to helping Iowa wounded, the citizens of Davenport had also requested that Archibald and the Relief Committee get the most accurate headcount of Iowa wounded possible under the circumstances. The chaotic nature of how the army handled the movement of its wounded down the Cumberland River made scurrying about from place to place an unfortunate necessity, if Archibald and the Relief Committee were to obtain an accurate count. With wounded scattered about in hospitals and hospital ships like so many white fluffy cottonwood seeds on a warm spring day, he and the Relief Committee made a habit of checking every hospital and hospital ship known to them, because they probably felt that it was the only way to complete the task. After having settled the color sergeant, Archibald intended to leave Mound City to check on hospital ships and hospitals down the Ohio River at Cairo and across the Mississippi River at Bird's Point. He wanted to gather information on wounded Iowa soldiers at these points, and where needed, render aid as he had done at Mound City. Events interfered with Archibald's plans.

Before he could leave Mound City, he received orders to "select all Iowa soldiers that could be moved without material danger and have them transferred to the steamer *T. J. Pattle*."[124] Mr. L. C. Burwell noted in his report that the Davenport

Relief Committee loaded "all of Cos B and C [Iowa 2nd Infantry] there were [at Mound City Hospital] and some others of the Iowa 2nd to the number of 16."[125] In short, the Davenport Relief Committee showed its vote of no confidence in the medical treatment at Mound City Hospital by moving as many Iowa soldiers as they could out of it. The Committee made sure that the wounded soldiers from the Davenport area (Company B and C of Iowa 2nd Infantry) got on the boat.

The intended destination, Cincinnati, was a much better place. As the home of a branch of the U.S. Sanitary Commission for the Valley of the Mississippi, the hospital there had good coordination and supply of medical assistance from the Commission.[126]

After the wounded were loaded on the boat, Archibald tried to resume his intended journey down the Ohio River to Cairo and Bird's Point. He did not intend to head up the Ohio River with the steamer ship loaded with wounded. Archibald left Mound City and went to Cairo. He checked on wounded Iowa soldiers on a hospital ship docked at Cairo that was on its way to hospitals in St. Louis.

After leaving that ship, he stood on Cairo's wharf hoping to catch another ship to Bird's Point in Missouri. Fate intervened to send him in a different direction. While Archibald stood on the wharf at Cairo, Mr. L. C. Burwell and the Captain of the *T. J. Pattle* surprised him.

Archibald expected Mr. L. C. Burwell and the *T. J. Pattle* to be going upriver to Cincinnati with all the wounded Iowa soldiers from Mound City. Instead, they had made a short trip downriver to Cairo, which was the opposite direction. Mr. L. C. Burwell explained in his account that he intended to pick up additional medical supplies that the Relief Committee had left at Cairo. According to Archibald, Mr. L. C. Burwell and the post surgeon in charge of the boat went looking for him in Cairo because they believed that they needed Archibald to help keep the wounded alive on the trip upriver.

Whether the meeting on the wharf at Cairo was by chance or design, Archibald found himself headed up the Ohio River with Mr. L. C. Burwell and the Iowa wounded on the *T. J. Pattle*. The post surgeon on the boat, Dr. Dunning, appointed Archibald first assistant surgeon and Mr. L. C. Burwell as ward master on the boat. As Mr. L. C. Burwell noted, these appointments "enabled [them] to do all that could be done for the Iowa boys."[127] Mr. L. C. Burwell also got Mrs. Magill, who had lent her room to H. B. Doolittle, assigned to the boat as a matron and cook. Mr. L. C. Burwell believed that if she had not accompanied them, then "the men would have suffered with hunger" on the five-day boat ride upriver to Cincinnati.[128] As it was, Archibald explained that the supplies on the boat were "very inferior and meager indeed."[129] Archibald praised the captain of the boat for providing "many privileges not in the bill" and also praised the aid from Davenport citizens that he and Mr. Burwell distributed to make up for the poor supplies provided by the army.[130]

By filling the gaps in the supplies, Archibald reported that he "succeeded in producing a marked improvement in every case under [his] care."[131] Another doctor on the boat was not so lucky and lost two men during the five-day trip. While no mention is made of the practices the other doctor used in treating his patients or the condition the patients were in when loaded, Archibald sought to assure the citizens of Davenport in his published report that the wounded transported had made it safely to Cincinnati.

The boat made frequent stops on the way up the Ohio River. At each stop, Archibald made every effort to collect information on the hospitals and any Iowa wounded located in them. He continued to work on getting an accurate count of wounded and sick Iowa soldiers and their locations. His diligent habit of gathering this information indicates how scarce and valuable such information on wounded soldiers' location and condition was at that time.

In their separate reports, Mr. L. C. Burwell and Archibald provided hints of their activities during the typical day on the boat loaded with wounded headed up the Ohio River. In all likelihood, Archibald, Mr. Burwell, and Mrs. Magill had a daily routine similar to the routine recorded by the Western Sanitary Commission in its report from one of its hospital boats during this part of the war. The routine was as follows:

> As soon as we got under way, the ladies set to work to wash and cleanse, and comb the hair of the sick and wounded. Warm water, soap, sponge, and flesh brushes were brought in requisition. Not only the face and neck, but hands and feet, and other parts of the body had to undergo the purifying process. After this, the surgeons ... proceeded to dress the wounds and other severe injuries of our patients, in which again we were materially aided by the ladies and gentlemen of our delegation. This process required three or four hours daily.
>
> The following was the daily routine. Early in the morning the ladies attended to ablutions and cleansing the patients. Breakfast

> was then served to them, after which a careful surgical and medical examination was gone through. Then came dinner, when they were waited on by all on board who could be spared from duty. After dinner, they were read to and entertained by conversation. At supper again, they had the attentions of all on board. After which we had singing of sacred or national hymns, reading the scriptures, and prayer.[132]

After five days of something similar to that routine, it is easy to understand the reason Archibald described it as "a most tedious and laborious trip."[133] Archibald, Mr. L. C. Burwell, and Mrs. Magill arrived in Cincinnati with their wounded at noon on Sunday, March 2, 1862. The U.S. Sanitary Commission and its local organization very efficiently unloaded the boat in two hours and moved them to a hospital in Cincinnati about one mile from the boat landing.

Archibald spoke with the doctors at the admitting hospital and arranged to have the wounded that had been in his care placed at a hospital on Third Street under the care of Dr. Murphy, a "Surgeon eminent in his profession," according to Archibald.[134] Because Archibald had practiced in Ohio for many years, it is possible that he knew Dr. Murphy and the other doctors in Cincinnati.

While Mr. L. C. Burwell reported in vague terms that the Cincinnati hospital conditions were much improved, Archibald beamed about the improved hospital conditions and the effect it had on the soldiers. Archibald explained that in a short time, the wounded were transported from the ship to "comfortable quarters surrounded by all the facilities usually found in the most improved hospitals and many luxuries that are not often found even there."[135] By luxuries, he meant good, nutritious food. When he visited the wounded in their new hospital in Cincinnati, he found them clean and in comfortable beds, in well-ventilated wards, with nurses and surgeons, and "regularly furnished with the best of food."[136]

The hospital conditions in Cincinnati stood in contrast to the deplorable conditions at Mound City. The hospital at Cincinnati had support from an active, very well-funded local sanitary society, and from the U.S. Sanitary Commission, which had a branch office located there.

The long days and hours laboring on the ship had caused Archibald to become severely ill. Mr. L. C. Burwell reported that Archibald was still sick on March 4th—three days after their arrival in Cincinnati. Archibald made no mention of his illness, which is unusual for him. He must have gotten somewhat better by March 5,

1862, because he and Mr. Burwell made the rounds to the hospitals to visit the wounded on Wednesday and Thursday of that week. On Friday, Mr. Burwell left to take a one-armed Iowa soldier to relatives in Ohio. Archibald advanced the funds for Mr. Burwell and the Iowa soldier's trip. On Saturday, March 8th, as Mr. Burwell's letter went to press in Davenport, Archibald accompanied two wounded Iowa soldiers on their return to Davenport. While he paid his way, the U.S. Sanitary Commission furnished the funds for the soldiers' return tickets. Archibald and the wounded soldiers returned to Davenport on Tuesday, March 11, 1862. After treating H. B. Doolittle, Judge Linderman also returned and reported that he was very unhappy with conditions in the Mound City Hospital.

Mr. L. C. Burwell's report credited the Davenport Relief Committee and other similar committees as critical to the delivery of necessary care for the wounded. In the Committee's view, the "Government had made no adequate preparations for an emergency like this."[137] His use of the word emergency is odd, because in a war, a battle is not an "emergency." Casualties in battle are an unfortunate outcome that to some measure should be anticipated. Mr. L. C. Burwell did not mean to disparage the army surgeons who were "unceasing in their labors."[138] He did mean to fault the army for terrible logistics. Mr. Burwell noted that when the committee left Mound City on February 26, 1862, the hospital there was out of bandages and hospital supplies. This only got worse in the next big engagement—Shiloh. Before Shiloh, Archibald and his fellow volunteers were about to learn the limits of public generosity for medical relief in early 1862.

CHAPTER 7: Mobilizing the Citizens to Support Soldiers' Aid in Davenport

Shortly after Archibald and the remainder of the Davenport Relief Committee returned to Davenport, the male citizens began serious efforts to formalize and sustain their sanitary affairs efforts for the duration of the war. The male citizens adopted a constitution for the Scott County Soldiers' Relief Association on April 8, 1862, and organized separate committees.[139] Scott County Soldiers' Relief Association appointed Archibald along with several other local doctors to the organization's surgical committee.[140] The Association inherited the earlier soldiers' relief activities that had begun at the February meeting in the Le Claire house.

The male citizens in Davenport woke up to the need for private citizens to provide soldiers' aid and medical assistance to the sick and wounded later than the women. The men's wives, sisters and daughters had already formed the Davenport Ladies Aid Society and the German Ladies Aid Society. Given their absence from Reverend Kynett's list of cooperating organizations, the inference is that the ladies aid organizations supported Annie Wittenmyer and the Keokuk Ladies Aid Society network.[141]

The founding of the male Scott County Soldiers' Relief Association was perhaps part of Reverend Kynett's strategy to exert greater control over the efforts to collect donations for soldiers' aid. The Iowa State Sanitary Commission needed to build its local donor base in existing population centers to compete with Annie Wittenmyer's Keokuk Ladies Aid Society network. The unorganized male population of Davenport and Scott County represented an opportunity for enlarging donations.

Despite holding potential as a base for donations, the Scott County Soldiers' Relief Association had an immediate shortage of cash in April 1862. By that time, the Association had exhausted the $784.20 in donations raised earlier in February 1862, on efforts to provide medical aid to Iowa soldiers after the Battle of Fort Donelson.[142] Before the members of the Davenport Relief Committee left in

February, the male citizens of Davenport had entrusted them with medical supplies and some of the cash funds raised for the effort. The members of the Relief Committee were led to believe that the expenses they incurred over and above the amounts entrusted would be reimbursed.

In April, the Association determined to resolve its funding and donation problem by establishing a systematic method to collect money and in-kind donations. The finance committee created a list of every male living in each ward and township of Scott County, using the existing ward and township system in Scott County. A finance committee representative or his assistant approached each man "above the age of 18 years" and recorded "the fact whether such persons do or do not contribute" and the amount of money or articles donated.[143] The Association also published in the *Davenport Daily Gazette* a request that ladies aid societies, the schools, and the benevolent societies donate "money, bandages, lint, hospital stores etc. to assist this Association in the important labor devolving upon it and also to render every possible assistance to the members of the Finance Committee in order that every household in Scott County may be solicited or have an opportunity to contribute." [144]

The finance committee's method relied on social pressure. By canvassing everyone and writing down donations, the social pressure to donate and contribute must have been fairly great, particularly in such as small setting. Those who failed to contribute risked ostracism and being associated with the anti-war Copperheads. Within a little over a week, the finance committee reported at April 17th meeting that they had collected $324.10 in new money.

The Association itself showed admirable transparency. It published its fully itemized list of income and expenditures connected with the Davenport Relief Committee's trip to Fort Donelson in the *Davenport Daily Gazette* on April 4, 1862.[145] The Association also clearly felt a duty to account for each dollar entrusted to it by the public including the funds that had been entrusted to the members of the Davenport Relief Committee on their February-March trip.

After returning, Archibald and Dr. McCarn submitted reports accounting their expenditures of money and supplies entrusted to them. However, the money provided by the Association had not covered all their costs. Accordingly, Archibald and Dr. McCarn sought reimbursement for their expenses from the finance committee at the end of March. They were not seeking compensation for their medical services that they had donated pro bono. [146]

To possibly forestall objections to their expense reimbursement requests, Archibald and other members of the Davenport Relief Committee submitted letters and reports on their activities to *Davenport Daily Gazette* for publication in March 1862. While the primary reason was to report news about the local soldiers and the committee's activities, a secondary reason was to explain the level of undertaking and possibly to build public support to repay the money that the committee members, like Archibald, had advanced. The reports also allowed Archibald and other Davenport Relief Committee members to document in a transparent way that they had used and distributed the money or goods given to them as instructed by the male citizens of Davenport.

Despite their efforts, a controversy over the expense reimbursements erupted. Archibald and Dr. McCarn received uneven results in their efforts to seek reimbursement from the finance committee.[147] Archibald sought reimbursement for funds that he had advanced on the Association's behalf to wounded soldiers for their travel on furlough. The committee approved and reimbursed Archibald's expenses. Dr. McCarn was not so lucky. The finance committee disapproved of how Dr. McCarn expended funds entrusted to him. In addition to denying his request for reimbursement, the finance committee requested that he refund to the committee $77.70, which was not a trivial sum.[148] Dr. McCarn defended his expenditures on behalf of a wounded soldier and for other members of the Relief Committee (Ira Gifford, Judge Linderman, and Mr. L. C. Burwell) who apparently had agreed to pay their own way before they left Davenport for Fort Donelson.

In the end, Dr. McCarn repaid $10.00 and received a public scolding by the finance committee through the newspaper for failing to expend $150.00 dollars in accordance with instructions.[149] While the finance committee probably believed that it looked responsible in protecting the public's donations, it looked cheap and petty in retrospect. The expenditures that Dr. McCarn submitted were for transportation costs of bona fide volunteers who participated in the activities that their citizens had requested of them. This was not the last time the Scott County Solders' Relief Association showed itself to be miserly. Their decision had negative consequences. The treatment of Dr. McCarn had an immediate effect on how future volunteers expended their own funds, because the prospect of being denied reimbursement for legitimate expenses was very real.

Just as the Association got itself organized, the Union Army under General Grant was surprised by General Johnston's Confederates at Shiloh Church near Pittsburg Landing on the Tennessee River. The Association met and determined to send another relief committee, including Mr. Burwell and Mr. Brown as nurses, and

Archibald and Dr. Gamble as surgeons. The surgical committee for the Association recommended that the Association compensate the nurses at the rate of $2.00 per day plus expenses and the surgeons at $100.00 per month. The Association's Executive Committee declined the compensation and offered only to reimburse the expenses.[150] Because the Relief Committee had already left, the Executive Committee sent a telegram informing the Relief Committee that they would work for free with only expenses paid. If they were unwilling to agree, they could return. The Relief Committee did not return.

The Association likely did not have the funds, or the ability at the time to raise funds, to pay expenses and to compensate the relief committee members. The Association had spent nearly all of the $784.20 it had initially raised in February and March on the expenses associated with the battle at Fort Donelson without providing any compensation. Given that the Battle at Shiloh Church, also called the Battle of Pittsburg Landing, looked to be a serious battle, they may have found it difficult to raise sufficient funds to cover salaries as well as expenses.

Besides, the Association had a bigger, more central concern: the construction of a hospital in Davenport for sick and wounded soldiers.[151] In April 1862, they began to organize a campaign for a hospital.

While the people of Davenport took initial steps to get a hospital sited there, the Relief Committee's focus was on the aftermath of the battle at Shiloh Church and its work to put the Iowa wounded on river transports bound for existing hospitals in the North.

CHAPTER 8:
Tending to the Fallen at Shiloh and Sending Them Home

While the Scott County Soldiers' Relief Association busied itself with a constitution and passed the hat for donations, the Union Army of the Tennessee under General Grant advanced south along the Tennessee River to Pittsburg Landing after the capture of Forts Henry and Donelson.

General Grant's Union Army of the Tennessee on Sunday morning held positions stretched between Owl Creek and Lick Creek on the bank of the Tennessee River around Pittsburg Landing. The topography around Pittsburg Landing where the Union Army sat was "undulating, heavily timbered with scattered clearings" and "considerable underbrush."[152] The broken, timbered ground inhibited visibility and communication, which played a part in the battle and complicated medical relief.

General Grant and his army waited there for the Union Army of the Ohio to join them in an assault on Corinth, Mississippi, where Confederate General Johnston was gathering his army. Corinth, Mississippi, stood on a key junction of several east–west railroads tying the Confederacy together.

On Sunday, April 6th, the Confederate Army attacked. With successive waves, they pushed the Union Army back toward the landing on the first day. On Monday April 7th, General Grant, with reinforcements from the Army of the Ohio, counterattacked and drove the Confederate Army back. In the fighting, the Union suffered 13,047 causalities, and the Confederates reported 10,699. Of the Union casualty total, over 8,000 were wounded. Also on Sunday, April 6th, General Prentiss and about 2,200 Union soldiers, many from Iowa, were captured when his division failed to fallback and the Confederates flanked his position on both sides.

The news of the Battle of Shiloh sent the Scott County Soldiers' Relief Association in full motion. It was reported that all the Iowa regiments in Grant's Army of the Tennessee had been engaged and likely had seen heavy casualties.[153]

Everyone was anxious. The new Relief Committee (Archibald, Dr. Gamble, Mr. Burwell, and Mr. Brown) was sent via railroad to Cairo on April 11th, a mere four days after the battle concluded.

As with the last Relief Committee, the members of this Relief Committee were charged by their fellow citizens to provide news and information on the Iowa soldiers to the public in Davenport. They did, sending reports for publication in the *Davenport Daily Gazette*. Dr. Gamble sent a letter early in the process on April 17, 1862.[154] Later, after the work of transferring many of wounded was finished, a Joint Physician Report from Archibald and Dr. Gamble was published on May 9, 1862.[155] Mr. Burwell, upon his return to Davenport in June, published his account.[156] Finally, after he returned in late June 1862, Archibald wrote a private letter report to Governor Kirkwood that touched on details not discussed elsewhere.[157]

Upon arriving at Cairo, Illinois on April 12, 1862, via railroad at 6:00 a.m., the Relief Committee, including Archibald, reported to Dr. Taggort, medical surveyor; General Strong, post commander; and Dr. Douglas of the U.S. Sanitary Commission. The Relief Committee explained its mission and sought permission to carry it out. Dr. Taggort offered Archibald and Dr. Gamble positions of surgeons in charge of rebel prisoners being transported to Columbus, Ohio. Archibald and Dr. Gamble declined.

At 8:00 a.m., the group headed over to the St. Charles Hotel in Cairo to meet with Governor Yates of Illinois and his surgeon general. The Committee requested their assistance. In summarizing the discussion and outcome, Archibald said that the consultation "resulted in many fair promises" from the governor of Illinois and the Illinois surgeon general, "but which promises were afterward studiously evaded by his Excellency and suit."[158] A Victorian way of saying the governor and his surgeon general made lots promises that they could not, or never intended to, make good on to help the Committee get to Pittsburg Landing.

After the fruitless meeting with the governor of Illinois, the Davenport Relief Committee along with others from Iowa met together to address assembling information on wounded and dead soldiers. Given the number of casualties, the Iowa relief volunteers, including the Davenport Relief Committee, were concerned that they might miss boats carrying Iowa wounded. To fill in this potential gap, the Iowa volunteers had a meeting that morning while at Cairo and chose Dr. Ennis to "remain and visit all hospital boats arriving at that point, and obtain all the names and destination and character of the wounds of such troops as were on board—this was done that none should be overlooked."[159] When they eventually moved up the

Ohio and Tennessee Rivers, the group stopped and made inquiries on all hospital boats, and "when opportunity offered, accurate lists of names, regiments, and casualties were made."[160]

By 9:00 a.m. on April 12, 1862, General Strong ordered the Relief Committee to go to Mound City Hospital to care for 700 wounded arriving from Pittsburg Landing. As the Davenport Relief Committee arrived in Mound City, Dr. Franklin and the Mound City Hospital were under investigation for alleged incompetent treatment of Iowa soldiers. Judge Wright of Iowa in April 1862 had brought a formal complaint against Dr. Franklin. In an April 11, 1862, letter to the War Department, Governor Kirkwood of Iowa pressed the matter. A formal investigation at the request of the U.S. Army surgeon general in April 14–15, 1862, cleared Dr. Franklin of the charges. Apparently, the investigation put the matter to rest.

There is no evidence Archibald or Dr. Gamble were involved in the investigation. Dr. Franklin appears to have held no outward malice toward the Iowa delegation despite the complaints. While at Mound City Hospital, Archibald and Dr. Gamble were offered positions as ward surgeons at the hospital, which they both declined. They instead proceeded to board the transport boat *City of Memphis*, which was carrying the wounded. On the boat, they "labored several hours in dressing wounded and supplying the immediate wants of" the roughly 70 Iowa soldiers on board.[161]

The Relief Committee portrayed in their reports the impression that they maintained an unerring focus on providing the aid to local Iowa wounded from the Battle of Shiloh at Pittsburg Landing. In their surgeons' report, Archibald and Dr. Gamble created the impression that like the ancient Greek Odysseus, they forged ever onward to their goal of gathering the Iowa wounded at Shiloh, to tend their wounds, and put them on a ship to a hospital. They kept their eye on the goal, despite numerous obstacles and distractions placed in their path, including the offer of paying positions. It must have been tempting to take appointments that paid real salaries, particularly when the Association had declined to offer any compensation and only to cover the Committee members' expenses. This was particularly true for Archibald, whose finances had not yet recovered from the financial crash of 1857. Archibald later felt the sting of his unpaid volunteering when, in the summer of 1862, his creditors foreclosed on his real estate investments for failure to pay debts due.

It is no doubt true that with limited resources and time, Archibald and members of the Relief Committee focused first on helping Iowa wounded. This was the same protocol used in the response to the battle at Fort Donelson. Because of the chaos after the battle, the administrators of the hospitals and medical wards were desperate for all the help that they could get, even if the assistance was given to only the wounded from a particular state.

After treating the wounded on the transport ship at Mound City, Dr. Gamble and Messrs. Brown and Burwell caught a steamer headed up the Tennessee River closer to the site of the recent battle. Archibald remained at the Mound City Hospital on Saturday, April 13th and Sunday, April 14th to "assist in several surgical operations."[162]

Dr. Gamble exited the steamer at Savannah, Tennessee, which is just down the river from Pittsburg Landing/Shiloh, on Sunday, April 14th. In Dr. Gamble's letter of April 17th, he reported that he found over 2,000 thousand wounded at Savannah. Dr. Gamble "for 48 hours dressed wounds" before he took the short journey upriver to reunite with the other members of the Davenport Relief Committee on Tuesday, April 16, 1862.

While Dr. Gamble and Archibald were temporarily detained, Messrs. Burwell and Brown proceeded straight to Pittsburg Landing (Shiloh) on Sunday, April 14th. There they met Mrs. Ann Harlan, the wife of Iowa's Senator Harlan, and Mrs. Annie Turner Wittenmyer, among others. They decided to work together to get the wounded and sick Iowa troops on a transport and sent north to a hospital, preferably in Iowa.

Upon arrival at the battle site on April 16th, Archibald and Dr. Gamble formed the opinion that the medical assistance provided by the surgeons at Shiloh had failed, in part due to the lack of proper medical supplies. In their May 9, 1862, report, they noted "the regular as well as the volunteer surgeons were seriously embarrassed in their efforts to relieve the wounded, by want of material to dress the wounds, and also the want of medicines and proper food for the sick. The preparation for the sick and wounded was very imperfect. They [the sick and wounded] were crowded into any and every place, without regard to location or comfort, and often left for days together without medical aid, or even common attentions of camp life."[163]

Archibald and Dr. Gamble accused the Army Medical Corps of failing not only in providing the needed medical supplies, but also in neglecting the wounded in scattered locations. Their observations are quite similar to those made by the U.S. Sanitary Committee in the Valley of Mississippi delegation, including Dr. Newberry, who arrived around the same time. Like Archibald and Dr. Gamble, Dr. Newberry reported finding at Savannah, Tennessee, "sick and wounded crowded into churches, dwelling-houses and structures of all kinds, filling to repletion every place at all fitted to hold them. The suffering and destitution were extreme."[164] Like Archibald and Dr. Gamble, Dr. Newberry in his report also noted that "the number of surgeons and nurses was entirely inadequate, and the resources of the Medical Department in the way of bedding, clothing, dressings, and diet, so exceedingly meager, that it is scarcely too much to say that all things necessary to the proper care of this great mass of suffering humanity were wholly wanting."[165]

If the scene at Savannah, Tennessee, was a disaster, the Pittsburg Landing battle site was worse. While Archibald and Dr. Gamble avoided describing the scene there, Dr. Newberry in his report noted that "the scene that met [his] eyes [at Pittsburg Landing] was one to which no description, though it exhausted all the resources of language, could do anything like justice."[166] In vivid detail, Dr. Newberry wrote that vast supplies of war and soldiers were being unloaded from ships at Pittsburg Landing in "wild and hopeless confusion. ... the wounded, borne on ambulances or on litters to the boats; the dead, lying stiff and stark on the wet ground, overrun with almost contemptuous indifference by the living; the busy squads of grave diggers rapidly consigning the corpses to the shallow trenches."[167]

The medical situation at Pittsburg Landing had been made worse by the manner in which the battle had played out.[168] Early in the engagement, the Union Army had been driven from its camp, which caused the loss of extensive medical supplies. Also, the desperate, chaotic situation of the first day with the lines pushed back to the river led to a fragmentation of the hospital system.

In fact, in a letter to Dr. Newberry of the U.S. Sanitary Commission, the Medical Director of the District of Ohio, R. Murray, revealed the depth of the U.S. Medical Corps' inadequate measures in his letter thanking the U.S. Sanitary Commission on May 8, 1862. Mr. Murray wrote "under the old organization of the Medical Corps of the army, [U.S. Sanitary Commission's boat] was indeed indispensable, and without it all the wants and comforts for sick and wounded could not have been met. At the same time, I must frankly say I consider it a great injustice to the Medical Corps of the army that, at the commencement of the present troubles, steps were not taken to place sufficient power, funds, and facilities at the disposal of the medical officers to enable them to provide for all the wants of the sick and wounded under all circumstances that could arise."[169] R. Murray's reflection ignores the Army Medical Corps' own failing to take the necessary actions and make the case to secure the necessary power, funds, and facilities at the beginning or at any moment up to the Battle of Shiloh.

Because of the terrible, chaotic conditions, the Relief Committee was determined to get the Iowa wounded away from the battle site as quickly as possible. They, however, needed a ship.

Mrs. Harlan, the wife of Iowa's Senator, was the savior of the hour. She secured the steamer *D. A. January* for the Relief Committee. As Mr. Burwell described it in his report, Mrs. Harlan "was the possessor of papers given in the handwriting of the Secretary of War, giving her such powers and privileges as clearly exhibited the great confidence he [Edwin Stanton] had in her integrity and ability to make proper use of the same."[170] Using the power granted by the Secretary of War, Mrs. Harlan had the *D.A. January* ordered to transport Iowa wounded to Keokuk, Iowa.

Curiously, Archibald and Dr. Gamble did not mention Mrs. Harlan's letter in their report. They instead indicated that the group met with Dr. Simons, medical director at the Shiloh battle site "and solicited and obtained transports."[171] Archibald and Dr. Gamble stated that "in our efforts to obtain transportation for the wounded, we were ably assisted by Annie Wittenmyer of Keokuk and Mrs. Senator Harlan of Iowa; also by our fellow citizen Hiram Price of Davenport and Mr. E. Clonky of Iowa."[172]

The U.S. government had purchased the *D. A. January* for use as a hospital steamer.[173] The Western Sanitary Commission in St. Louis had fitted it out, and Surgeon A. H. Hoff of U.S. Volunteers was in charge of the boat. When the news of Battle of Pittsburg Landing (Shiloh) had come, General Halleck requested the Western Sanitary Commission to send hospital boats, including the *D. A. January*. Because of the *D. A. January*'s connection to the Western Sanitary Commission, it is possible that Annie Wittenmyer's connections to that group also were instrumental in securing it for use in transportation, which is why Archibald and Dr. Gamble credited her efforts as well as Mrs. Harlan's efforts in securing the *D.A. January* for their use.

On Tuesday, April 16th, the Relief Committee reunited. Over the sixteenth and seventeenth, the Committee finished collecting the Iowa wounded at Pittsburg Landing (Shiloh) to be loaded on the *D. A. January* for transport. Mr. Brown and Mr. Burwell had been laboring to collect the wounded there since Monday the 15th. Dr.

Gamble in his letter of April 17th conveyed the sheer enormity of this task when he noted that the wounded "extended over a region of five miles."[174] While at Pittsburg Landing, Archibald and Dr. Gamble visited several Iowa regiments, collecting names of the wounded still in the field at Pittsburg Landing and information on wounded that had already been sent north.

After loading as many wounded as they could find at Pittsburg Landing, the Relief Committee moved downriver to Savannah, Tennessee, on Wednesday, April 17th, with the *D. A. January* just a few miles downriver. They loaded all that they could locate at Savannah, Tennessee, except about 100 Iowa wounded. After the loading was finished on April 19th, the *D. A. January* left with Mr. Burwell, Mrs. Harlan, and Annie Wittenmyer bound for the hospital in Keokuk, Iowa.[175]

Around about April 17th, Archibald received "from Adjutant General Baker a communication, requiring myself and Dr. Jas. Gamble as Surgeons to proceed to St. Louis."[176] He ignored the order. Instead, he and Dr. Gamble determined that they could do the most good by staying near the battlefield at Shiloh, where there was evident suffering. Archibald did not want to completely ignore the order from Nathaniel Baker, Adjutant General of Iowa. To protect himself and Dr. Gamble, Archibald reported to a different Iowa State official, Iowa Surgeon General Hughes, and asked Surgeon General Hughes to clarify if remaining at the battlefield was inconsistent with the purpose of the mission. Archibald got no reply and so persisted to do what he thought he should do—treat the wounded at Shiloh and its surrounding areas like Savannah, Tennessee.

While at Savannah, tragedy struck on the night of Saturday, April 19, 1862. The Relief Committee, including Archibald, met on the steamer *Dunlaith* with members of the Wisconsin delegation, including Wisconsin Governor Harvey. These two groups sought to discuss "the best plans for accomplishing [their] humane mission."[177] While Archibald makes no specific mention of Annie Wittenmyer, she was there.[178] Archibald reported that the steamer *Hiawatha* approached the steamer *Dunlaith* to come alongside. Governor Harvey stepped out of the *Dunlaith*'s cabin and attempted to board the *Hiawatha*. He intended to request passage for the Wisconsin delegation. He missed his step and fell in the Tennessee River.

Archibald said, "A moment after, we were startled by the cry of 'A man overboard.'"[179] The group attempted "prompt and heroic efforts" to give Governor Harvey assistance, but "in the extreme darkness of the night, the rapid current, and amidst steamboats and barges all proved useless."[180] The governor of Wisconsin drowned.[181]

The sudden and tragic death of the governor likely influenced one of the primary recommendations made by Archibald and Dr. Gamble in their report. Archibald and Dr. Gamble recommended against, "States and Cities sending large delegations calculated to interfere with the operations of the army near the scene of the conflict."[182] Archibald called that "worse than useless." It was an indictment of the relief committee system that he had already participated in twice.

Instead, Archibald and Dr. Gamble recommended that the state of Iowa appoint agents to be with the army at post hospitals. These agents of the state would "take charge of sanitary goods, and be on hand and ready at all times to render immediate and efficient aid to [Iowa] forces in the field and to the sick and wounded in the battle."[183] These agents were to report back to the people of Iowa on the conditions, needs, and wants of the soldiers.

In that recommendation, Archibald and Dr. Gamble advanced the idea of creating an Iowa state sanitary agent or agents, which the Iowa Legislature would eventually pass into law later in 1862. Archibald and Dr. Gamble envisioned these agents distributing timely aid "after the battle" and before the wounded moved to a hospital upstream "when assistance is most needed—immediate and efficient aid then would save hundreds of lives."[184] These were needs that the U.S. Army had demonstrated, up to that time, it was incapable of meeting.

In their report, Archibald and Dr. Gamble also noted the schism between the surgeons of the volunteer regiments and the surgeons of the regular army. The regular army surgeons "obstructed at almost every step by official arrogance and egotism" the work of the Relief Committee. The regular army physicians generally were critical of volunteer surgeons and civilian surgeons like Archibald.[185] The Relief Committee, by contrast, had nothing but nice things to say about the surgeons for the volunteer regiments.

As an additional recommendation, Archibald addressed the lack of dedicated transport for wounded troops. Securing transport could have been a serious problem, because without Mrs. Harlan's letter, it is not clear that they would have gotten a transport. The members of the Relief Committee did not have a transport with them when they arrived. The state of Iowa, unlike other states, had not sent a transport at state expense. Dr. Gamble in his letter of April 17th and Archibald in the Joint Surgeon's Report highlighted the state of Iowa's failure to provide a transport and recommended the state consider finding funds to acquire and fit out its own ship. In retrospect, this was a case of assuming that the present conditions would continue, but the steamer ship proved to be not necessary as the battlefront changed and other organizations filled this niche. Archibald's letter calling for a hospital boat led the state authorities to empower the next governor's agent, Ira Gifford, to "charter a steamboat on the Tennessee for the conveyance of wounded soldiers home or to hospitals" if Colonel Ira Gifford deemed it necessary.[186]

Later, Archibald changed his mind about a state hospital boat, at least officially, and stated that no boat was needed.[187] Ira Gifford, in his letter, made clear that "Dr. Maxwell" joined in his recommendations, including the one on hospital boats. Archibald's retraction may have come because he had noticed the progression of the war made a boat unnecessary by that time. Also, the idea may have belonged to Dr. Gamble, since it first appeared in his letter on April 17th.

In their May 7th report, Archibald and Dr. Gamble did not pass up the opportunity to stress the suffering and expense that they had endured on behalf of the citizens of Davenport. While travelling on boats, they had to furnish their own provisions and bedding. When on land, they travelled through drenching rains and deep mud. At night, they slept on the ground, with only a thin blanket for covering. When they did stay at an inn, "the charges were enormous, and the fare most miserable."[188]

Given that Archibald and the others expected the Association to reimburse their expenses, the description of the conditions and expenses incurred were likely made with the view to improving the chances that their reimbursement submission, which accompanied their report, would be approved. Because Dr. McCarn's expenses after Fort Donelson had been denied and the Association had rejected salaries, it made good sense to stress the hardships and costs encountered, reducing the likelihood of any challenge to reimbursement.

The fear that the Scott County Soldiers' Relief Association would not reimburse had a negative effect on the use of goods meant for the soldiers. In fact, Archibald said, that he "expended but little money save for board and travel expenses."[189] His frugality stemmed from "the fact that [he] used in all cases when [he] could get them, sanitary supplies of soldiers."[190] The stinginess of the Association likely led Archibald to use supplies meant for soldiers instead of spending money that might not be reimbursed. Given that Archibald's financial situation was not good and that he had volunteered for several months, he likely had no intention of advancing significant amounts of his own funds only to face the same trouble that Dr. McCarn had with his Fort Donelson expenses that April.

Despite the hardships, Archibald said that he and his companions "did not regret their hard fare, as midst it all, many were the cheering evidences of kind appreciation received from the suffering soldiers."[191] Also, the doctors had received "many gentlemanly courtesies tendered them by the surgeons of the volunteer regiments."[192] This contrasted with the treatment from surgeons of the regular army from which Archibald and Dr. Gamble did not feel that they had received any gentlemanly courtesies.

Archibald and Dr. Gamble remained near Savannah, Tennessee, after the *D. A. January* left with Annie Wittenmyer, Mrs. Harlan, and Mr. L. C. Burwell on April 19–20th. The two also sent Mr. Brown, who was ill, home on the *Hiawatha*, the boat that the late governor of Wisconsin tried to board. On April 24th, they journeyed south to Pittsburg Landing (Shiloh). They learned that the remnants of three Iowa regiments (8th, 12th and 14th) had been combined into a Union brigade. These regiments had suffered significant losses at the Battle at Shiloh in men captured, killed, and wounded. The day after, on April 25th, Archibald and Dr. Gamble borrowed horses and rode out to visit and check on the health of more distant Iowa regiments.

On April 26th, Archibald traveled north alone back down the Tennessee River to Savannah. That day, Dr. Gamble and Archibald parted ways because Dr. Gamble accepted an offer to join the Iowa 3rd Infantry Regiment as its contact surgeon. Archibald returned to Savannah to continue moving wounded north. He reported that he "succeeded by politeness of Dr. Woods of Cincinnati, in getting on, in comfortable quarters, all of Iowa's sick and wounded" fit to travel from Savannah on the steamer *Tycoon*.[193] The *Tycoon* was one of two first class steamers that the Cincinnati Branch of the U.S. Sanitary Commission had provided for use in transporting wounded from the battlefield at Pittsburg Landing (Shiloh).[194]

Having sent many of the Iowa wounded home on steamers in April, Dr. Gamble and Archibald began considering their options for remaining with the army as surgeons. The army's regular surgeons had made it difficult for the two men to provide medical services, probably because Archibald and Dr. Gamble's association with a local Iowa organization did not command respect. This likely prompted Dr. Gamble to accept the contract surgeon appointment for the Iowa 3rd Regiment. As April 1862 came to a close, Archibald went into the employ of the state of Iowa and reported to Surgeon General of Iowa Dr. Hughes. During this time, Archibald was given the rank of regimental surgeon and reported directly to Major General Halleck's Chief Medical Officer Dr. Simons.

After the Battle of Shiloh, Major General Halleck took command, making General Grant his second in command.[195] By the end of April, General Halleck was ready to advance the 19 to 20 miles southwest to attack the strategic town of Corinth, Mississippi, where a Confederate Army under Generals Van Dorn and Beauregard waited. To advance on Corinth, General Halleck united about 120,000 men in the three Union Armies: the Army of the Ohio under General Buell, the Army of the Tennessee under General Thomas, and the Army of the Mississippi under General Pope.[196] Corinth lay at the intersection of the Memphis and Charleston Railroad and the Mobile and Ohio Railroad. When the Union captured Corinth, it severed the Memphis-Charleston railroad a key artery tying the eastern Confederate states to the western states.

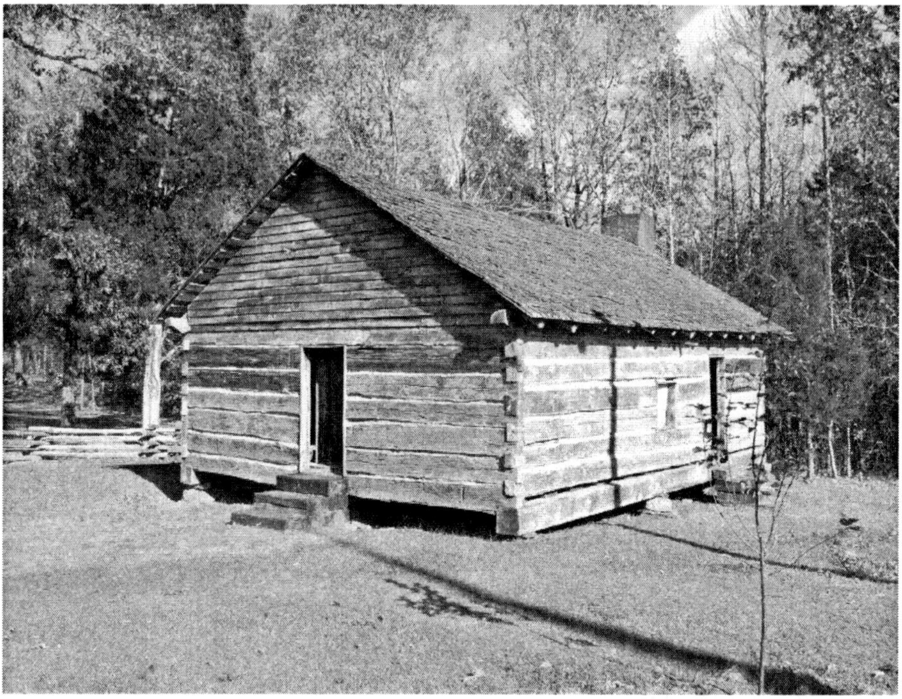

A replica of Shiloh Church at the Shiloh Battlefield Park in Tennessee. Picture provided with permission courtesy of Mary Christenson.

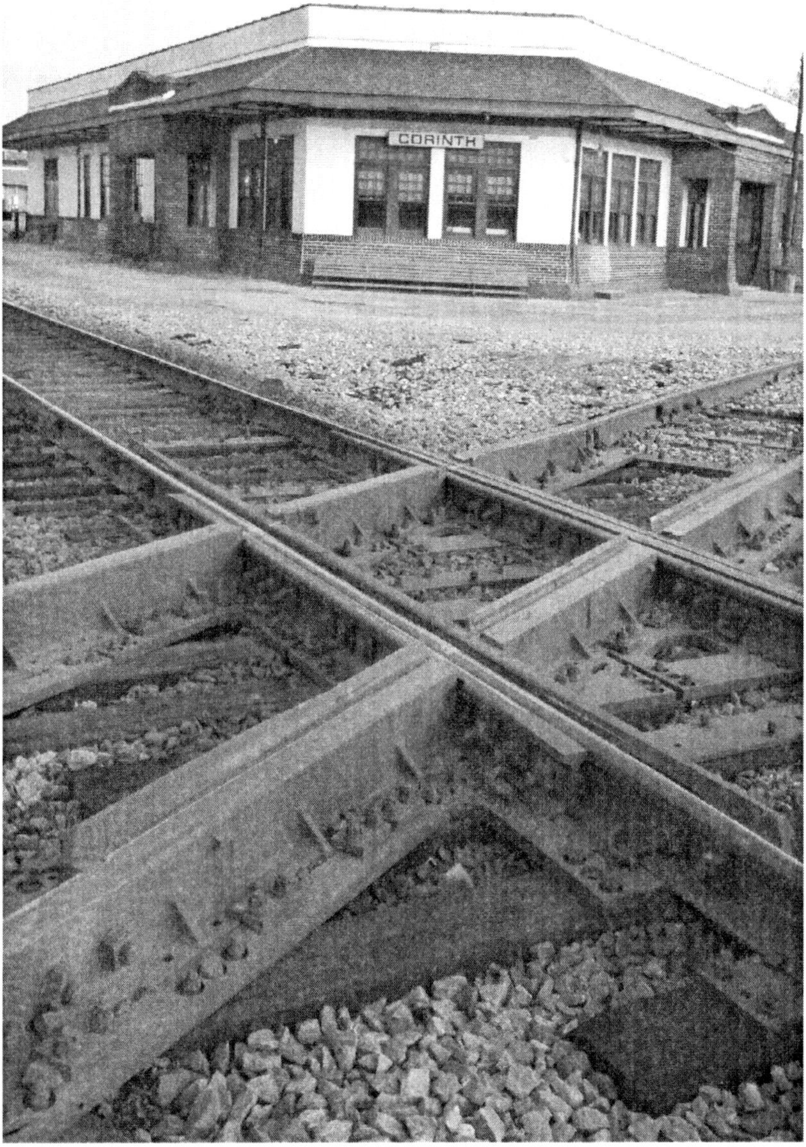

The Memphis-Charleston and Ohio-Mobile Railroad Crossing in Corinth, Mississippi. Picture provided with permission courtesy of Mary Christenson.

CHAPTER 9:
Regimental Surgeon in the Advance on Corinth

On May 1, 1862, Archibald received orders from Adjutant General Baker of Iowa to stay in the Hamburg-Pittsburg landing area and to coordinate the transfer of Iowa wounded soldiers to northern hospitals. Another battle was anticipated. The three, united Union Armies advanced on Corinth slowly. The medical department prepared for the potential battle that might follow. At the time, Archibald, as a regimental surgeon reporting to Dr. McDougal, worked in a variety of roles. In those roles, he focused mainly on treating Iowa sick and wounded.

During his time at the Hospital in Hamburg, Archibald and others on the Committee continued to act as news reporters in addition to fulfilling their medical duties. They took upon themselves to report the news from the front. Archibald was particularly prolific and forwarded reports and letters to the *Davenport Daily Gazette* reporting on his activities on May 8th, 9th, 14th, 19th, and 26th, and in a private letter to the governor of Iowa on June 30, 1862. Ira Gifford and Mr. L. C. Burwell also published reports during the same period.

Archibald had a hand in establishing the hospital at Hamburg. On May 1, 1862, Archibald, with Dr. McDougal of the U.S. Sanitary Commission, went to Hamburg, Tennessee, to establish a hospital for convalescing soldiers. Later, Post Surgeon Dr. Varian took over for Dr. McDougal at Hamburg, and Archibald continued to assist Dr. Varian in establishing the hospital. Dr. Varian and Dr. McDougal drew upon the U.S. Sanitary Commission's stores to establish the hospital and a supply depot for the Corinth Campaign in early May at Hamburg, Tennessee, six miles north of Pittsburg Landing on the Tennessee River.[197] By the beginning of May, Archibald reported that by his count, 600 Iowa soldiers out of a total of 3,700 wounded were admitted in the hospital in Hamburg.[198]

Dr. Varian assigned Archibald as the surgeon in charge of the 8th Ward at the Hamburg Hospital. Archibald expressed it a little differently in his letter from May 7th, stating that he "consented to be assigned, for the present, to the 8th Ward" of the Hamburg Hospital, as if he had choice.[199] In the 8th Ward, he had 160 wounded and sick men from a number of Iowa regiments. He continued to remain as the surgeon in charge of the 8th Ward as the number of wounded increased during the assault on Corinth. By the time he wrote his next published letter from Hamburg Hospital on May 11th, he was caring for 200 wounded in his 8th Ward, and the hospital had almost 4,000 and expected it to get only worse.[200] He noted at the time that he was "making every preparation to meet the increasing demands."[201]

During his time as surgeon in charge of the Hamburg Hospital's 8th Ward, Archibald demonstrated excellent skill in keeping his wounded alive despite adverse conditions. Archibald reported on May 7th that he had lost none under his care. On May 19, 1862, Ira Gifford, the newly appointed Iowa State Agent, complimented Archibald, stating, "The Iowa boys and all others find sure relief from Dr. Maxwell. He is untiring in his efforts to help them and so far has been very successful—not having lost a man."[202] Archibald's track record continued at Hamburg until he left his post on May 19th for another position. In his parting letter, he mentioned that he had "lost none put under [his] care, although [he] had treated 700."[203] In treating his sick, Archibald had an advantage in that he drew upon the stores of the U.S. Sanitary Commission to ensure that his wounded and sick received better and healthier food.

Archibald experienced firsthand the difference it made to work in a U.S. Sanitary Commission hospital and near a U.S. Sanitary Commission depot, and he praised the U.S. Sanitary Commission. He said, "Sanitary Commissions are the salvation of the army."[204] Archibald was "delighted with the management of the U.S. Sanitary Commission."[205] Archibald valued the U.S. Sanitary Commission because its depot provided "all of his delicacies such as fruits, butter, lemons, liquor, clothing" that he got by requisition.[206] In fact, Archibald was frustrated because, while he took advantage of the stores, "many of the regiments [did] not get the benefit of this arrangement from the neglect of their surgeons."[207] Archibald encouraged the other surgeons to "get the Iowa regiments to send promptly to Dr. Douglas [the U.S. Sanitary Commission's doctor in charge of operations at Pittsburg Landing] and get the benefit of [U.S. Sanitary Commission] supplies."[208] By the time Ira Gifford arrived, Archibald had succeeded in making requests for U.S. Sanitary Commission supplies by Iowa regimental surgeons more customary.

Archibald remained fixed upon food and preparing it in a manner that was edible for the wounded. In his letter on May 7th, he wrote, "have nurses plenty, but need good cooks." He repeated his plea in his May 11th letter, "good cooks are needed very much."[209] He told Iowa State Agent Ira Gifford in May 1862, to have people from Iowa send pepper sauce and "soda crackers and butter and anything of a nourishing nature."[210] Archibald's complaint for better food was an old one. He had made similar observations in reports after the battle at Fort Donelson in February 1862. In fact, he continued to raise this issue throughout his service.

Meanwhile the Union Army advanced on Corinth very slowly. Archibald estimated in his May 7th letter that the Army advanced three miles a day. This is consistent with General Grant's account in his memoirs. General Grant explained that General Halleck had the Union right wing, the Army of the Tennessee (which General Grant was nominally in charge of), and the Union center, Army of the Ohio, advance slowly, building roads and entrenchment lines as they moved forward. General Pope with the Union Army of the Mississippi on the Union left was more aggressive, but General Halleck ordered him to pullback on multiple occasions slowing the advance on Corinth.

General Halleck sought to avoid another battle like Shiloh. Archibald and many others believed that the strategy would force a siege of Corinth. In his May 11th letter, Archibald said, "there are few points, either north or south, where nature and improvements (railroads, etc.) have done more to complete a strong military position for defense than this same Corinth, and our friends need not be alarmed if they should learn that a siege be the only course to effect their [the Confederate's] defeat."[211]

On May 8th, General Pope and the Union left wing had made aggressive movements on Farmington, Mississippi, which is not far from Corinth, Mississippi. As a result, the Iowa 2nd Cavalry saw heavy engagement. In his May 11, 1862, letter, Archibald penned the details on the Iowa 2nd Cavalry wounded and killed in action at Farmington. Archibald explained that in the advance on Corinth via Farmington, the Iowa 2nd Cavalry had charged a Confederate battery to provide time for a Union brigade under General Paine to retreat. The most severely wounded remained in the hospital camp in Tennessee consistent with General Halleck's orders.

Archibald also mentioned in his May 11th note that the *D. A. January* had just left, transporting some of the Iowa 2nd Cavalry wounded home. Throughout May 1862, the *D. A. January* made multiple trips, carrying mainly Iowa wounded between the Pittsburg Landing area in Tennessee back to the hospital in Keokuk and other northern hospitals.[212] Archibald, as a surgeon at the hospital at Hamburg, assisted in the effort. Mrs. Harlan and Mr. Burwell continued to work loading the wounded on the *D. A. January*. They continued to focus on moving only Iowa wounded, which was not unusual, as similar groups from other states did the same for their citizens, much to the chagrin of more national organizations like the U.S. Sanitary Commission.[213]

Archibald and the Iowa delegation's effort to spirit their wounded north was a standard practice by other state and national delegations, including the U.S. Sanitary Commission. General Grant and other Union generals were highly critical of the practice of sending all the wounded that could be transported north and away from the battlefield, because it put lightly wounded soldiers far away from their units and delayed the time that they could be put back into the fight.[214] By Vicksburg, this practice had changed.

Shipping wounded north for treatment had other supporters besides Archibald. Dr. Newberry of the U.S. Sanitary Commission defended shipping of all the wounded out of Pittsburg Landing area because the Hamburg-Savannah-Pittsburg Landing area had become ridden with disease. Dr. Newberry noted in tones that sound hyperbolic but capture his view that "the pestilential atmosphere of the country about Shiloh was producing an amount of sickness almost without parallel in the history of war." [215] Because in Dr. Newberry's view "the sick required to be removed to a healthier locality before recovery could take place," it was best for the hospital steamers to take them to hospitals in the north.[216] In Dr. Newberry's opinion, the transport of the 7,000 wounded "saved the army and the country a great number of lives."[217] He lamented that "if all the sick of the army before Corinth had been taken from the deadly atmosphere that enveloped camps and hospitals, there would have been more brave men in our ranks in subsequent battles; more living, loving fathers and husbands in happy homes at the North; fewer mounds in the soldiers' cemeteries, and fewer pensions paid to widows and orphans." [218]

By his May 11th letter, Archibald felt left behind. He wrote that he "had received no instructions or sanitary goods from [Mr. Russell] or any other person in Iowa, although [he] had again and again reported to [Mr. Russell], Reverend Kynett, [and] Dr. Hughes."[219] He provided his address in his published letter so that supplies or instructions might be sent. Likely on May 11th, Archibald did not realize that Colonel Gifford had been appointed state agent by the governor of Iowa at a May 7th meeting. He also did not know that Ira Gifford and Mr. L. J. Center had been sent along with supplies to Pittsburg Landing to check in on Archibald.[220]

Archibald had not been forgotten. Quite the contrary, Governor Kirkwood had secured for him an appointment on the medical staff of General Pope, commander of the Army of the Mississippi, which made up the left wing of the Army advancing on Corinth. Reverend Kynett and Mr. Russell, the corresponding secretary of the Scott County Soldiers' Relief Association, had suggested the appointment to the governor. On May 19th, Archibald received his orders to report to the headquarters of Major General Pope immediately.

When he left the hospital on that day, Archibald felt that he was leaving things in good hands. He fixed "up affairs of the ward."[221] He was most happy to have Ira Gifford's assistance, reporting in his letter that "a great load has been lifted off my [Archibald's] shoulders—I feel that I can now have one on whom I can rely for aid and counsel."[222] Mr. L. J Center was busy with the sick as Archibald prepared to leave for the front lines of the left wing under General Pope.

When Archibald reported to General Pope's Headquarters on May 19, 1862, he was "assigned duty on the advance in his division where [he] was to give particular service" to the 10th Iowa Infantry Regiment and also a number of other Iowa infantry regiments and the Iowa 2nd Cavalry, which made up a brigade.[223] According to the note sent by the assistant surgeon for the Iowa 10th Infantry, Archibald served as surgeon of the 10th Infantry Regiment from May 20th until June 12th.[224] During this time period, General Pope, along with the rest of Union Army, advanced on Corinth. On May 26, 1862, Archibald witnessed a "sharp skirmish in which the 10th Iowa led by Col. Perczal behaved gallantly."[225]

On May 26th, unbeknownst the Union Army, the Confederate General Beauregard had published his order to evacuate Corinth by May 29th. Trains began to evacuate the Confederates and their war material from the city as the Union Army under Halleck approached, seemingly without noticing the evacuation. General Halleck drew his army up in contemplation of a siege. On May 30, 1862, Union troops entered Corinth without the expected battle or siege to find the enemy and supplies gone.

General Pope and his Army of the Mississippi were sent in pursuit of the retreating Confederates. General Buell with the Army of the Ohio followed them. Archibald, along with the 10th, advanced until coming to a halt at Burnsville. Archibald reported that the "health of portions of the army was considerably affected by the forced marches they [had] undertaken. . . .The water, too, was often execrable." [226]

On June 10th, General Pope and his column returned and fell back into camps near Corinth. At the time he left, Archibald did not believe that the Army of the Mississippi would be leaving the Corinth area for some time.[227] He happened to be right about that.

Archibald used the expected window of inactivity and his ill health as an excuse to return home to Davenport in June 1862. In fact, Archibald was so sick that he refused to wait around to provide his medical assistance on a steamer with wounded bound for a hospital in the north. Publicly, he reported that he was ill due to his "unremitting exertions among the sick."[228] In a private letter to the Governor, he explained that his health had broken down "by experiences incident to the advance" after the retreating Confederate Army, when he rode 20 miles a day and drank terrible water. He was back in Davenport by June 19th, feeble and with impaired health. He rested 11 days before writing Governor Kirkwood his report.

CHAPTER 10: The Rivalry Continues—Sanitary Affairs on the Home Front

Archibald's return home brought him back into the center of the political rivalry between Annie Wittenmyer soldiers' aid organization and Reverend Kynett's organization. By May–June 1862, Archibald found himself fully caught in its net, particularly over efforts to make the two organizations work together. In early 1862, Mrs. Wittenmyer had set out terms, in a letter to the governor, under which the Keokuk Ladies Aid Society network might cooperate with Reverend Kynett's Iowa State Army Sanitary Commission. Based on her subsequent actions, she meant work together in their joint effort. She never intended to dissolve her network of ladies aid societies across Iowa. In contrast, Reverend Kynett wanted her and her network of ladies aid societies throughout the state to submit to his authority and work through him.

Annie Wittenmyer continued to build on her reputation. She provided needed aid at the front and personally delivered sanitary supplies to the Iowa soldiers. She spoke with the soldiers and surgeons at the front and in the frontline hospitals about their needs. Armed with that knowledge, she returned to Iowa to raise the needed donations. At the same time in early 1862, she sought out connections and authorizations to assist her in her task. Her impeccable connections included a friendship with General Grant and his wife, which allowed her to operate with minimal hindrance. Her authorizations included a letter from Secretary of War Edwin Stanton that permitted free travel and shipment of sanitary supplies.

Despite Annie Wittenmyer's progress, Reverend Kynett continued to press for the union of the two networks under his management. Annie Wittenmyer's network pushed back with another scathing letter published in the Iowa newspapers. In an April 1862, the Keokuk Ladies Aid Society attacked Reverend Kynett's Iowa State Sanitary Commission as woefully ineffective at delivering its aid, because the Iowa State Sanitary Commission's collected goods sat in a warehouse and had not been delivered to the field.[229]

In May 1862, Reverend Kynett sought to address the criticism and assert control. First, Reverend Kynett attempted to remedy the supply distribution problem with the governor's appointment of Colonel Ira Gifford as State Agent in the field. After his appointment in May 1862, Colonel Gifford made trips carrying supplies to Iowa regiments at the front. But, Reverend Kynett found it impossible to control Colonel Gifford, and his instrument eventually turned on him. Second, a Relief Society convention was called in Davenport on May 28th in an attempt to more permanently address the problem with the supply distribution in the field and to attempt to force the Keokuk Ladies Aid Society network to submit to Reverend Kynett. Third, the Relief Society convention was meant to lend legitimacy to the Iowa State Army Sanitary Commission by having citizens from all the counties in Iowa appear to support it.

Reverend Kynett's hand was in the selection and appointment of Colonel Gifford, even though it was done under the umbrella of the Scott County Soldiers' Relief Association. The published minutes of the May 7, 1862, Executive Committee meeting for the Scott County Soldiers' Relief Association reported that the Society needed an agent in the field to provide information and "a faithful disposal of all supplies donated."[230] Because the group already had Mr. Burwell and Dr. Maxwell in the field providing reports, someone was needed to distribute the supplies. The organization "deputed Reverend A. J. Kynett to act for them, and through him (Reverend Kynett), a commission (from Governor Kirkwood) was secured for Colonel Gifford as agent of the State with authority to visit sick and wounded in the field and render them assistance as may be needed."[231]

Ira Gifford arrived at the front in May with supplies to distribute. It also appeared that Ira Gifford was on a mission to make sure that Archibald supported the aims of the May convention. He sought out Archibald soon after arrival and sent a letter that was published two days before the convention.[232] Among the recommendations in the letter, Ira Gifford wrote:

> "I would recommend—and Dr. Maxwell joins me herein—the organization of a Relief Society at the Convention called for on the 28th inst. (May) to be known as a branch of the United States Sanitary Commission, and that they call upon all relief societies and sanitary committees to come together and act in harmony and do away with all petty jealousy. The societies already formed need not

> disband, but resolve to send their supplies to one fountainhead, and they will in that way have the same voice and representation, and will be entitled to an agent in the U.S. Commission who being an Iowa man will see that Iowa soldiers do not suffer."[233]

The political purpose of the endorsement was to show that Archibald supported Reverend Kynett's vision for the Iowa State Sanitary Commission as an auxiliary to the U.S. Sanitary Commission and that all local Iowa soldiers' relief organizations should submit to his authority. By May 1862, Archibald had become well known for his service in sanitary affairs. He had been selected twice by the male citizens to go on the relief trips and had several published reports of his efforts in the local newspaper. Also, the Scott County Soldiers' Relief Association had listened and heeded many of his recommendations after Shiloh.

Additionally, people began to take notice of the valuable medical assistance Archibald provided at the front, which probably added weight to his recommendation. As a sign of how highly his services were valued, Reverend Kynett and other leading men in Iowa politics from the Davenport area wrote to the governor stating that Colonel Gifford's report corroborated, "accounts previously received from various quarters of the skill, industry, and faithfulness with which Dr. A. S. Maxwell of this city [Davenport] has labored and is still laboring among the sick and wounded at Pittsburg Landing and vicinity."[234] Additionally, Hiram Price, Treasurer of the Iowa State Sanitary Commission and a leader in the Iowa Republican Party reported to Governor Kirkwood, "I have no hesitation in saying that Dr. Maxwell has rendered very faithful efficient Service during his absence [from Davenport]. All who return from the field of his labors that I have seen bear testimony to his usefulness and indeed I doubt if there are many physicians who have rendered the service which he has."[235]

In giving his endorsement of the May convention, Archibald probably understood the political and practical value that came with supporting Reverend Kynett and the rest of the Iowa State Sanitary Commission. Archibald continued to search for a more permanent appointment in the army, and recommendations were very important in securing such positions. At the time, Reverend Kynett appeared to have the ear of the governor. Before and after the endorsement, Reverend Kynett interceded on Archibald's behalf. First, he interceded with the governor to assist with Archibald's appointment on General Pope's medical staff in May 1862. After the appointment to Pope's medical staff, Reverend Kynett and his group of worthies again requested that "the surgical department of our army would be benefited and our state honored by the appointment of Dr. A. S. Maxwell as Brigade Surgeon to some one of the Iowa brigades now in the field."[236] Later when Dr. Maxwell returned from the field in ill health, Reverend Kynett interceded with another letter to Governor Kirkwood, requesting that Dr. Maxwell be considered for post surgeon at the Davenport Hospital to be constructed.[237] At the same time, Iowa State Army Sanitary Commission Treasurer Hiram Price also pressed the governor to "have [Dr. Maxwell] appointed one of the 40 additional surgeons recently allowed the army."[238]

With Archibald and Colonel Gifford's endorsement, the State Soldiers' Relief Convention kicked off in Davenport on May 28th at Le Claire Hall in the morning and moved to the Methodist Church in the afternoon. The *Davenport Daily Gazette* reported on the convention in the newspaper the next day. The convention was a male-only affair, which was odd given the prominence and importance of the ladies aid societies. In fact, future conventions on the topic did not repeat this oddity. The convention did attempt to gather support for building a hospital on the Mississippi north of Keokuk.

The real purpose of the May 1862 convention was to legitimize Reverend Kynett's Iowa State Sanitary Commission by having male citizens from across the state recognize it as the one official state organization. At the end of the morning, the convention adopted a motion that the "members of the State Sanitary Commission represent the state at large."[239] The convention claimed to have representatives from each of the Iowa counties to vote on matters, giving it the appearance of conferring a statewide people's mandate in its pronouncements.

Reverend Kynett sought to legitimatize the governor's original request that Annie Wittenmyer's Keokuk Ladies Aid Society and its network submit to his authority along with all other local soldiers' aid societies in the state of Iowa. Toward the end of the convention, he introduced the following resolution, which the convention adopted:

> Resolved, that the several County Soldiers' Relief Associations and Ladies Aid Societies, now organized, or hereafter to be organized, be and are, hereby, requested to report to the State Sanitary Commission, unless they have already done so, their several organizations, including date of organization, and list of officers and post office address.[240]

Reverend Kynett directed his resolution at the group of organizations that had not submitted to his authority—the Keokuk Ladies Aid Society network.

The convention also adopted resolutions to encourage the creation of local soldiers' relief organizations subordinate to the Iowa State Sanitary Commission. With the Keokuk Ladies Aid Society sending their donations and goods through a different channel, the pressure was on Reverend Kynett's Iowa State Sanitary Commission to increase its donation base. The creation of new groups provided the Iowa State Sanitary Commission with new avenues to generate donations of goods and cash. Reverend Kynett's organization never did manage to get the Keokuk Ladies Aid Society network to send their goods through him to the U.S. Sanitary Commission, but he never ceased trying to cut them out or break them up. The convention was just another lever.

Reverend Kynett also attempted to have the convention address the criticism leveled by the Keokuk Ladies Aid Society against the Iowa State Sanitary Commission in the April 1862 article that the donated goods had not been distributed. Even prior to the convention, Colonel Gifford had passed along in his report published in the *Davenport Daily Gazette* that May the remark from the U.S. Sanitary Commission representative at Shiloh, Dr. Douglas, that the U. S. Sanitary Commission had distributed more goods from Boston to Iowa soldiers than the Commission had received from Iowa. Attempting to remedy this deficiency, the delegates adopted a resolution calling for a state agent in the field "to look after the health and general welfare of Iowa soldiers."[241] The state agent, who at the time of convention was Colonel Gifford, was instructed to "communicate to the Iowa State Army Sanitary Commission (Reverend Kynett) what particular kind of supplies are needed and to what point the same shall be sent."[242] Upon receiving the request, Reverend Kynett was obligated to send supplies as requested. With this process set up, Reverend Kynett and his Iowa State Sanitary Commission hoped to avoid future accusations that the donations were being left unused in warehouses in St. Louis. Also, through the state agent in the field, Reverend Kynett no doubt hoped to make Annie Wittenmyer appear redundant.

Even if he could not make Mrs. Wittenmyer redundant, Reverend Kynett attempted to extend an olive branch for cooperation (under his terms, of course) to the Keokuk Ladies Aid Society network. The convention adopted a resolution "that nothing contained in the foregoing resolutions is intended to interfere with the several Ladies Aid Societies, but on the contrary we cheerfully acknowledge the very valuable assistance already received from the patriotic ladies of Iowa and hereby earnestly invite their continued aid in this good work."[243] The need to adopt such a resolution demonstrates their fear of another public letter from the ladies aid societies embarrassing Reverend Kynett and the Iowa State Army Sanitary

Commission. However, it also ominously attempted to mask the structural changes that Reverend Kynett hoped to bring about to alter the dynamic and force a union.

With the May convention concluded, Reverend Kynett and the Iowa State Sanitary Commission may have appeared strengthened with the public endorsement. Nevertheless, it was not long before cracks appeared in the façade.

While Reverend Kynett may have thought he had politically outmaneuvered Mrs. Wittenmyer on the home front, he had vastly underestimated her ability to turn the tables on him by convincing key public supporters Ira Gifford and Archibald that she and her methods were superior to his. In Davenport and in the public realm, Reverend Kynett's own handpicked state agent, Colonel Gifford, who was supposed to offset Annie Wittenmyer's rising notoriety, gave Annie Wittenmyer a huge endorsement in his report published in the newspaper on July 1, 1862. The endorsement hit the papers on the eve of a second co-ed soldiers' relief meeting in Davenport. Colonel Gifford wrote,

> ...I met with Mrs. Annie Wittenmyer, General Agent for the Ladies Aid Society of Keokuk, Iowa. She had just arrived from St. Louis, with a large quantity of choice stores, seventy-five boxes in all. This lady has been indefatigable in her exertions for more than a year, and in all her movements a model of industry, zeal and propriety. With a keen perception of what is necessary to be done, and will to execute that never admits the word "fail" into her vocabulary, combined with the suavity of a high-toned and educated woman, she moves in her sphere easily and gracefully, and overcomes obstacles which those of the sterner sex could scarcely hope to surmount. The soldiers of Iowa, who have been suffering from wounds and diseases, owe to this excellent and thorough-going person, a debt of gratitude, which should entitle her always to a generous and cordial welcome to every patriotic hearth-stone within the bounds of the State. Mrs. Wittenmyer was able to furnish to the regiments of Iowa a large quantity of stores, and in a matter of distribution, I cooperated with her to the best of my ability.[244]

Colonel Gifford's eloquent and fulsome praise for Annie Wittenmyer was an endorsement of her and the Keokuk Ladies Aid Society network for donation and distribution of aid. His report confirmed that donations to Annie Wittenmyer's organization did make it to the Iowa soldiers' hands. He also made plain that Annie Wittenmyer would do what it took to see that the Iowa soldiers received the aid.

Reverend Kynett could not tell such a story, because he was not taking the supplies to the soldiers at the front like Annie Wittenmyer. The Iowa State Sanitary Commission's model relied on shipping to the U.S. Sanitary Commission for general distribution, which painted a less colorful picture.

The May convention had barely been over a month when Annie Wittenmyer came to Davenport to take up the offer of cooperation offered in the May convention. In doing so, the political winds shifted in her favor. The *Davenport Daily Gazette* reported on July 3rd that Mrs. Annie Wittenmyer had arrived intending to remain only a few days. Notice for a meeting of Soldiers' Aid Societies at 9:00 a.m. on that day circulated in the *Davenport Daily Gazette*.[245]

As advertised, the meeting began at 9:00 a.m. in the Christian Chapel in Davenport. The members of Davenport Ladies Aid Society attended in support of Annie Wittenmyer. The executive committee for Scott County Soldiers' Relief Association supported Reverend Kynett, along with "as many of the different aid societies, and the public generally."[246] On the July 3rd morning, the two opposing groups elected Archibald president of the joint meeting.

At the joint meeting, Annie Wittenmyer put her offer of cooperation on the table. The *Davenport Daily Gazette* summarized her opening statement to the attendees. The purpose of her trip to Davenport was to "secure concentrated effort for the benefit of" sick and wounded Iowa soldiers.[247] She noted that Iowa had "a number of organizations in the State all working for the same object, but lacking unity of effort." She reportedly wanted a plan of cooperation with Reverend Kynett's group and suggested that "there ought to be somebody with the army to have some official character who would, in cooperation with [her], look after the welfare of" Iowa troops and see that the supplies sent to troops actually reached the troops.[248] She stressed the urgency of her concerns because of the rise in sickness in the Army at Corinth. Archibald agreed with her.[249]

In her proposal, Annie Wittenmyer also supported another key plank of the May convention—a call for an official state agent. However, she framed her offer in a way that preserved her and her network's independence. The state agent was to work with her and be her co-equal to share the load. By adopting the planks of the May convention on her own terms, she at once was supportive and yet preserved her and her organization's independence.

In addition to the issues of cooperation between the two rival sanitary organizations, the public voiced frustrations that the Army was slow to establish a hospital. Reverend Kynett defended himself and the Iowa State Sanitary Commission against an accusation that the Commission had worked "against Davenport." Even Annie Wittenmyer stepped up to defend him, although in defending him, she pinned him and his organization as the non-cooperator. According to the newspaper editor, Annie Wittenmyer said, "The Sanitary Commission had not co-operated with the Aid Societies as heartily as [I] could have wished, but [I have] heard of no feeling on its part against Davenport."[250]

The meeting concluded with the adoption of several resolutions related to cooperation. The first resolution thanked Annie Wittenmyer for "the energy and devotedness with which she has labored as the almoner of these societies in distributing hospital supplies and caring for the suffering."[251] The joint endorsement of both sides of the aisle showed that a large section of the populace supported Annie Wittenmyer's efforts and wanted her to continue.

The group also adopted Annie Wittenmyer's call for a state agent. A smaller committee was formed to meet and confer with her "as to the best plan to be adopted to secure a unity of action by the various aid societies of the State to ensure a systematic supply of sanitary stores and proper care of sick and wounded soldiers from Iowa."[252] In a blow to his control, Reverend Kynett was not appointed as member of that committee. It basically excluded him from discussion of the details of the cooperation going forward.

In a sign of unity, the two groups published in newspapers in August 1862 a circular announcing the union of their efforts.[253] The directions in the circular provided an address for individuals wishing to forward donations and goods to Reverend Kynett's organization, and a different address for people who wanted to donate to her organization care of Mrs. Knowles, who had become Corresponding Secretary of the Keokuk Ladies Aid Society. Annie Wittenmyer signed the circular, Special Agent Iowa Sanitary Association.

While the meeting led by Archibald did not go well for Reverend Kynett, he did not at first hold it against Archibald. In a letter on July 7th, Reverend Kynett again asked Governor Kirkwood to appoint Archibald to a different position as a chief surgeon.[254] Nevertheless, Archibald appears to have paid a price for supporting Annie Wittenmyer in the July meeting, because the record of Reverend Kynett and his worthies soliciting positions for Archibald dried up shortly thereafter.

The *Davenport Daily Gazette* on Monday July 7, 1862, carried a report from the committee on their meeting with Annie Wittenmyer. They determined that the appointment of a state agent by the governor was the best way to achieve Annie Wittenmyer's proposed plan of cooperation. The committee decided to send two delegates and Annie Wittenmyer to Governor Kirkwood to request that he appoint a state agent to "assist" her in "attending the sanitary condition of the Iowa soldiers and in sending them to hospitals near Iowa."[255] Annie Wittenmyer and the two delegates journeyed to Governor Kirkwood' s home in Iowa City, which was covered in an article in the *Davenport Daily Gazette* on Tuesday, July 8, 1862.

At that meeting, Governor Kirkwood complimented Annie Wittenmyer on her efforts. He expressed hearty support for her request. He commented that because the state had not had an agent at the front to send wounded and sick soldiers home, Iowa soldiers lay in hospitals scattered "like driftwood along the sides of an overflowed stream" along the route of march.[256] According to Governor Kirkwood, the state of Iowa had already incurred nearly $1,000 dollars in transportation costs to move Iowa soldiers back to Iowa from far-flung hospitals, an expense that might have been avoided if a state agent had coordinated efforts to send the wounded and sick to hospitals closer to Iowa.

As Annie Wittenmyer concluded her whirlwind lobbying effort for a state agent, Archibald suffered a blow to his personal financial stability. His inability to pay his debts became self-evident when a notice of foreclosure and sheriff sale on a quarter section and five town lots owned by him and Samuel Saddorris ran on the front page of the *Davenport Daily Gazette* on July 8, 1862.[257] The proceeds of the sale were to pay a debt of $874.97 owed to Lorenzo Schrieker. The foreclosure notice would run for many days.

No doubt, his largely unpaid service at the front had severely cut into his finances. In response to Archibald's June 30th letter to the Governor on his activities, Governor Kirkwood wrote on the back of Archibald's report on July 7, 1862, "[Hiram] Price at Davenport to have Dr. Maxwell paid $311.62 at the rate of $138 a month." Archibald must have labored even at the end of July under the impression that he had provided his services without pay based on the report compiled by Colonel Gifford, who passed along that tidbit in his report to the governor.[258]

Despite the financial distress, Archibald carried on with his work in service of the sick and wounded soldiers. He and a group of distinguished gentlemen took Dr. Barker on an inspection tour of the Davenport hospital that the Scott County Soldiers' Relief Association had established at Camp McClellan. Dr. Barker reportedly found the hospital to be "just the place, and ... was surprised that patients had not previously been sent there."[259]

Dr. Barker's remarks must have been sweet music to the ears of the Davenport hospital supporters. The Scott County Soldiers' Relief Association's report explaining its expenses and activities documented the time, effort, and expense that the organization had put into the establishment of the hospital. In fact, the report made clear that the Association's treasury was empty. An unpaid debt of $592.55 was due and unpaid related to the hospital.

Shortly after the inspection, Archibald prepared to leave the state again with Colonel Gifford. Archibald had recovered from his illness in June and now felt the need to return to provide medical assistance to the soldiers. While Archibald's financial situation troubled him, he remained committed to doing the great work to which he and others had been called—relieving the sick and wounded soldiers.

CHAPTER 11:
On a Ship Downriver with Colonel Ira Gifford

After the fall of Corinth, the Union Army made successive gains in Western Tennessee. On June 6, 1862, the Union captured Memphis, Tennessee, bringing the Mississippi River down to that point under Union control. With the earlier capture of New Orleans and Baton Rouge in Louisiana, Vicksburg and Port Hudson were the only significant Mississippi River towns still in Confederate possession. The railroad line in Vicksburg provided the only major line connecting the Confederate states west of the Mississippi River with the east. By dividing the Confederate states west of the Mississippi River from the east and cutting the railroads used to ship goods from the west to the east, the Union hoped to starve the Confederate's war machine of the material and men to sustain its effort in the field.

On July 11, General Halleck moved to Washington to take command of all armies. General Grant took his place in command of the Union army at Corinth, and General Sherman was in command at Memphis.

Ira Gifford prepared for a short visit to the front in Corinth to carry sanitary supplies and check on the Iowa regiments there. On or about July 12, 1862, Archibald expressed to Colonel Ira Gifford a desire to return to the front for an extended period of time.[260] Colonel Gifford gladly accepted Archibald's offer and asked him to take sanitary supplies to General Curtis' troops at Helena, Arkansas, before Archibald rejoined the army in Corinth, Mississippi. Colonel Gifford and Archibald planned to journey down the Mississippi River together to Memphis before they parted ways. Because Colonel Gifford was now working actively with Annie Wittenmyer, he explained his plans to Annie Wittenmyer in a July 12th letter, four days before his departure to enable them to coordinate their efforts.

Due to sickness in the family, Archibald missed catching the steamship with Colonel Gifford on July 16th out of Davenport to return to the front.[261] Archibald left later, catching a steamer to Keokuk, Iowa, where he planned to meet up with

Colonel Gifford. However, by the time Archibald arrived, Colonel Gifford had already left for St. Louis.

Archibald remained in Keokuk a while longer to take his medical board examination. Governor Kirkwood had likely arranged for Archibald's medical examination to make him eligible for a commissioned assistant surgeon or surgeon position in the army. Earlier in the month, on July 7, 1862, Mr. Saunder, a Davenport acquaintance of Governor Kirkwood, had written the governor on Archibald's behalf, communicating that Archibald was willing to take the examination. Mr. Saunder had indicated that Archibald was "fully aware of the position which a man can assume by being an assistant or a full surgeon. The latter would be his choice; the former [Mr. Saunder doubted] his acceptance of."[262] Mr. Saunder boldly asserted that Archibald was "entitled by his [accomplishments] as a medical man and his zeal in the great cause in which we all feel so deep an interest to at least [an appointment as a regimental surgeon]." Colonel Gifford conferred with the governor about available positions as well.

The medical examination for a Union Army surgeon, or assistant surgeon, commission was a new requirement in the Union Army. Surgeon General Hammond, a young reformer, had instituted it to ensure surgeons possessed minimum skills. Surgeon General Hammond required that doctors and surgeons pass a medical board examination before receiving a federal commission.[263] The examinations involved one to two hours on history, geography, zoology, literature, natural philosophy, and languages, and then a three-hour examination followed by seven or eight questions about surgery, anatomy, practice of medicine, pathology, physiology, obstetrics, medical jurisprudence, toxicology, materia medica, chemistry, and hygiene.

Archibald's exam was administered by Professor J. C. Hughes, M.D., who was head of the Keokuk College of Physicians and Surgeons. At the time, Dr. Hughes was also the Surgeon General for the state of Iowa and the head of the Keokuk Army General Hospital. Archibald passed. Upon hearing of Archibald's success, Ira Gifford proudly reported to Governor Kirkwood in his July 23, 1862, letter that Archibald passed his medical exam.[264] Apparently, not everyone who sat for the medical board passed in the summer of 1862.[265] Ira Gifford forwarded along a comment from Professor Hughes that Archibald "had met with the fullest approval."[266] Within three months of his examination, Archibald received a federal commission as an Assistant Surgeon at the Keokuk Hospital, and also the Chair for Pathology and Physiology at the College of Physicians and Surgeons in Keokuk.

Archibald and Ira Gifford met up in St. Louis on July 20, 1862. The next day, on July 21st, Archibald and Ira Gifford visited paroled Iowa soldiers who were confined at Benton Barracks in St. Louis until released from their parole.[267] These Iowa soldiers had been captured at Shiloh by the Confederates and had to wait in camp until they were formally exchanged for captured Confederate soldiers. After their exchange, the Iowa soldiers could return to their regiments in the field.

Archibald and Ira Gifford found the troops in a "most unsatisfactory state of mind."[268] The parolees had to sit around and wait. Also, the Union's "failure of promises that they should receive their pay" played a significant role in their state of mind.[269] In a letter to Annie Wittenmyer, Ira Gifford observed that while the Iowa soldiers were well supplied, they were upset and "disregarded all orders and were leaving camp at will in squads of from 10 to 20 in number. Some had been arrested and confined in irons."[270] Problems with parolees of this nature were not uncommon.

Archibald surveyed the scene of mass insubordination and intervened to get the soldiers to stop. According to Ira Gifford, Archibald "made a speech to them, which had a very good effect."[271] Archibald advised "them to return to the duty required of them," which was to sit in camp and wait to be exchanged so they could return to the field.[272] Archibald and Ira Gifford, in consultation with the general in charge at the barracks, wrote Governor Kirkwood about the missing pay and recommended the transfer of the most troublesome parolees.

After their visit to Benton Barracks, Ira Gifford and Archibald obtained passes to go downriver from St. Louis. Archibald and Ira Gifford purchased "potatoes and onions" for Archibald to take to General Curtis' Union Army at Helena, Arkansas.[273] Ira Gifford was bringing supplies to the Iowa regiments at Corinth, Mississippi, from the U.S. Sanitary Commission supply depot in Columbus, Kentucky. They both boarded the *G. W. Graham* steamer to head downriver at 6:00 p.m. on July 23, 1862, from St. Louis toward Memphis.[274] While on board, Ira Gifford wrote letters to Governor Kirkwood and Annie Wittenmyer.

After the Battle of Shiloh, the Union Army still was not taking steps to supply proper, nutritious food to keep its troops healthy. The Union Army ration was not unusual for its time. Nevertheless, the U.S. Sanitary Commission and the state sanitary commissions recognized that the troops needed more and better vegetables. They had to step in to fill the gap, because the Union Army either could not or would not. Ira Gifford and Archibald were essentially bringing vegetables to supplement the usual army fieldfare that generally consisted of salt pork or salt beef, beans, hard tack, and coffee.[275]

Ira Gifford may also have been sending Archibald to check on General Curtis' Union Army at Helena, Arkansas, because there was a report of a famine and scurvy in the army stationed there.[276] While in St. Louis, Ira Gifford visited with Mr. Yeatman, a commissioner with the Western Sanitary Commission, about the state of General Curtis' army. Mr. Yeatman assured him that the Western Sanitary Commission had kept General Curtis' army in "fine condition." Despite Mr. Yeatman's assurances, Archibald kept his plan to take potatoes and onions down the Mississippi River to the Union Army at Helena, probably out of caution.

After a brief stop at Cairo on Wednesday, July 24th, they proceeded onward down the Mississippi River to Columbus, Kentucky, where Union soldiers held the town. Columbus had been selected as the U.S. Sanitary Commission's base for supplies after the fall of Corinth because Columbus was connected to Corinth by railroad.[277] In Columbus, Ira Gifford and Archibald checked in with U.S. Sanitary Commission and obtained sanitary supplies for the trip.

Although well to the rear of the front lines, Columbus was not completely safe. Prior to their arrival, Archibald reported that Confederate cavalry had raided into Kentucky. The raiders had boldly ridden up under the Union guns defending Columbus and made the residents in some of the homes prepare them dinner.[278] Archibald was likely reporting on a cavalry raid by Confederate Colonel John Hunt Morgan.

Having avoided the Confederate raiders in Columbus, Ira Gifford and Archibald left for Memphis, Tennessee down the Mississippi River. On the way from Columbus to Memphis, their boat passed Island No. 10. While Island No. 10 had fallen earlier in the year to Union General Pope, Confederate raiders harassed Union shipping by setting cannon on riverbanks on either side of the island to shoot at passing ships. This apparently happened to Archibald and Ira Gifford's boat. Ira Gifford reported that "we were apprehensive of being fired upon from the banks of the river, but fortunately escaped the unwelcome visitation of a cannonball, though not so much could be said of the boat that immediately preceded us."[279]

Although they dodged the Confederate cannonball, Archibald and Ira Gifford encountered several passengers on the steamer who supported the Confederacy and were not shy about it. Archibald wrote of one such woman and her young boy named Jeff Davis, after the President of the Confederacy. Archibald said, the lady "discoursed quite freely on the way, etc. and at length when near me spread on her secesh doctrines rather thick. I stopped and looked in her face with an expression that must have denoted the surprise I felt that any rational woman should hold such sentiments in this country. She blushed, hesitated, sank back into her chair and turning to her little son who was repeating her sentiments said, 'That will do.' I heard no more secesh from that source."[280] Ira Gifford, in his letter, to Annie Wittenmyer on July 26, 1862, reported a similar encounter on the boat.

Archibald's encounter appears to have been not much different than a similar verbal altercation that Annie Wittenmyer had with a Confederate lady sympathizer in Nashville, Tennessee, after the fall of Nashville in 1862. The conversation that she had with the woman remained vivid enough that she was able to record it years later in her memoir *Under the Guns*. At the time, Annie Wittenmyer had checked herself into a hotel whose guests included supporters of the Confederacy. According to Annie Wittenmyer, the confrontation went as follows:

> I had no purpose of controversy in my heart; and so when the lady said, "My baby is named after the best man in the world, Beauregard." I only smiled.
>
> "I suppose you Yankees think you can conquer us?"
>
> "That is what the people of North hope to do."
>
> "Well you can't. There is not men enough in the North to conquer us; for when you kill the men off, the women will take up arms."
>
> "Well madam, there are thousands of men gathering and drilling in the North, and they will soon be here; and it's their fixed purpose to maintain the Union, cost what it will."
>
> "They will kill women will they?"
>
> "They will *conquer the South*."
>
> "Contemptible hirelings! They'll kill the women, will they?" She hissed.
>
> "I don't think they want to kill the women; but if that is necessary for the maintenance of the Union, I suppose they will have to do it."

> "Wretches! Wretches! They'll kill the women, will they?" She screamed, and her eyes blazed fire and scintillated like the eyes of a maniac. I thought she was going to leap upon me in her fury. We were standing facing each other; and I made up my mind that if she did assault me, that I would do my little share of fighting, and choke a little of the treason out of her. But she changed her mind and rushed from the room.[281]

Archibald and his contemporaries Annie Wittenmyer and Ira Gifford held firm convictions that the Union must not be allowed to fail. They did not tolerate the secessionist views in the South that they believed to be treasonous. It is not surprising that Annie Wittenmyer, Ira Gifford, and Archibald recorded these encounters in Tennessee within a reasonably short period of time after the Union Army had taken portions of states that had left the Union. It is doubtful that this was the last such encounter in their adventures with individuals openly supporting the Southern cause, but it may have been their first.

Having kept the Confederate ladies' opinions at bay, Archibald and Ira Gifford arrived in Memphis, Tennessee, at about midnight on July 25th. When they arrived in town, Archibald estimated that Union General Sherman had 12,500 to 15,000 Union troops under his command.[282]

In Memphis that day, Archibald and Ira Gifford observed freed former slaves "making fine defenses" for the Union Army. Archibald reported that the sight of the freed slaves "almost made me shout in the streets."[283] Ira Gifford's telling was equally enthusiastic, writing that the freed slaves were "happy as lords and free as the air. God be praised."[284] While many in the North did agree with Archibald and Ira Gifford's sentiments, freeing the slaves had not yet become a goal of the war for the North, as Lincoln's emancipation proclamation would not be issued until later in the year.

Later, Archibald took time that day to visit the beautiful city of 45,000. He claimed that he had "been all over the city; delightful place, but the people look sour."[285] Memphis had recently been taken by the Union, which likely explained the sour looks. Also, Archibald never passed up a moment to comment on the food. He said, there were "plenty of peaches in the market" but "hotel fare [was] poor and dear."[286]

On July 25th, Archibald and Ira Gifford went a mile and half outside of town to inspect the health of two Iowa regiments that were part of Sherman's forces there: the Iowa 3rd and 6th Infantry Regiments. The Iowa 3rd Infantry Regiment had just completed a 45 mile march from La Grange in 100-degree heat with insufficient water.[287] Ira Gifford and Archibald's inspection of the Iowa 3rd Infantry allowed for a temporary reunion with Dr. Gamble, who had worked with Archibald at Shiloh. Despite the long march, Archibald reported that the regiment was "in good health and spirits."[288]

After concluding their business with the two Iowa regiments in Memphis, Ira Gifford and Archibald loaded ten barrels of potatoes and onions on the steamer *White Cloud* destined for the Union Army in Helena, Arkansas. Ira Gifford then bid "God-speed to Doctor Maxwell at 7 o'clock in the evening" of July 25th as Archibald journeyed down the Mississippi River.[289]

Archibald's trip to General Curtis' army in Helena was very brief. By Friday August 1st, Archibald met up with Ira Gifford in Corinth, Mississippi.[290] In the intervening six days, he dropped off his supplies at Helena, checked on the Union soldiers, and went back up the Mississippi River, probably to Columbus, Kentucky. From Columbus, he took the train to Corinth, Mississippi.[291] Having completed the run to Helena, Archibald once again took a position similar to the one that he held prior to his departure from the Union Army in June.[292]

CHAPTER 12:
Battles and Skirmishes Around Corinth and in Sanitary Affairs

Having completed his run of sanitary supplies to Helena, Arkansas, Archibald met up with Ira Gifford outside Corinth, Mississippi. He rested and then went on a hospital inspection on August 3rd. Ira Gifford and he travelled about a mile and half south of Corinth to a spot where the army was in the process of setting up a general hospital.

Archibald and Ira Gifford did not like what they found at this field hospital. They found 700 patients "huddled in a few tents without any adequate preparation for their comfort and many of them past recovery."[293] Archibald diagnosed "quite a number of cases of scurvy."[294] Based on his inspection, Archibald concluded that "sickness is evidently on the increase, and is more fatal." The deplorable conditions and the scurvy moved Archibald, Ira Gifford, and the other many sanitary affairs and soldiers' relief organizations into action.[295]

To remedy the scurvy, Archibald implored people to send vegetables and butter. Vegetables at Corinth he wrote could not "be got at any price."[296] This was not unusual, as the armies on both sides of the conflict foraged for food. Archibald pleaded, "Friends at home should see that these veterans of many battles are not left to die for want of articles so plenty and cheap with them."[297] To further efforts to gather vegetables, Archibald had his August 11th letter from Corinth, Mississippi, making the case for the increased need for vegetables published in the *Davenport Daily Gazette* on August 16th in addition to providing basic information on sickness in two local Iowa regiments stationed at Corinth.

Ira Gifford returned to Iowa for the special purpose of collecting the much-needed vegetables. He left on August 6th with the plan of collecting vegetables to bring in early September. Archibald, as planned, stayed behind to provide medical assistance in the field.

When Archibald rejoined the Union Army of the Tennessee in August 1862, he found the Union Army troops scattered in small clumps trying to hold the hard-won territory in Western Tennessee and Northern Mississippi with a precariously fragile and inadequate route for supply and communications. For his friends and readers at home, Archibald wrote that "our troops are mostly 'laying around loose' all over this broken country—in small commands—depending principally on their supplies being brought by the Columbus Railroad [that] every day demonstrates its incapacity to meet this potential demand; even now we are on short rations of most important articles of substance."[298] Given the dependence on the one Columbus Railroad, Archibald and others with him were worried that, if the communications are "cut off—not an improbable occurrence—[then] great suffering among our troops would necessarily follow: For this country could not feed this army three days."[299]

Archibald had keenly perceived the Army of the Tennessee's strategic malaise that had descended upon it after General Halleck's departure and the departure of the Army of the Ohio to chase Confederate General Bragg in Kentucky. Archibald was not the only one concerned by the strategic situation. General Grant was "most anxious" because he was trying to hold the territory gained by the fall of Corinth and Memphis with but a fraction of the great army that had been used to capture it. A force of 35,000 to 40,000 Confederates under General Van Dorn prowled about looking to take advantage of the situation by capturing supply depots and cutting the Columbus Railroad lifeline. In fact on August 22, 1862, the Union garrison at Clarksville, Tennessee, surrendered.

Despite the strategic uncertainty, Archibald decided to stay. He took another contractual regimental surgeon position with the 13th Iowa Infantry Regiment stationed near Bolivar, Tennessee. Bolivar, Tennessee is a little town south and east of Memphis between Memphis and Corinth. The town lay along the defensive perimeter that General Grant set up to defend against the Confederate Army that probed his positions and cut off his main resupply route.

On August 30, 1862, the Union troops holding Bolivar, Tennessee, including Archibald and the Iowa 13th Infantry, found themselves in a lively action. A force of roughly 4,000 Confederates made a probing attack. After the skirmish, Archibald wrote a series of letters home to assure his wife and children that he was doing fine.[300]

At the time of the battle, the Union Army of the Tennessee's lines of communication back to the home front were so bad that Archibald's letters became breaking news about the fight, adding critical detail to sparse telegraph messages. The local newspaper picked them up and published them. In his letters, Archibald gave an eyewitness, detailed account of a skirmish.[301] As Archibald related the action, two Ohio infantry regiments and an Illinois cavalry regiment marched out to engage the attacking Confederates. During the battle, Thompson's Indiana artillery advanced to support the three Union regiments in the field. The 13th Iowa Infantry Regiment was ordered out at 11:00 am to support the artillery, but was not heavily engaged. The Union forces eventually fell back to "within a mile and half of Bolivar" and then were ordered back to quarters.[302]

Archibald wrote letters home to reassure people that he was "well, and so far, comparatively safe."[303] The troops had dug fortifications. The Union forces were "in good condition to defend themselves," although he believed that they were "nearly surrounded by a superior force."[304] Archibald also noted that the Confederate forces' probe of Bolivar, Tennessee, was part of a series of such attacks on the railroad between Bolivar and Jackson, Tennessee.

While bullets flew on the battlefield and casualties mounted, tensions built up at home in Iowa sanitary affairs. Ira Gifford, Annie Wittenmyer, and Archibald had worked together to create a unified Iowa State Sanitary Affairs effort to address the sanitary and relief needs of the troops. Ira Gifford arranged for vegetables and other sanitary relief supplies that he had gathered and sent to Annie Wittenmyer through the U.S. Sanitary Commission's Columbus, Kentucky, depot.[305] Ira Gifford expressed his intention to return to the field and "in concert carry on our noble work with an energy to ensure the relief to Iowa's sons so much needed."[306] For his part, Archibald coordinated with Annie Wittenmyer on distribution of sanitary goods at the front and also looked after the nurses' health.

However, not everyone was happy to cooperate. By the time Ira Gifford had returned to Iowa in mid-August to gather much-needed vegetables and other supplies, Reverend Kynett had begun to strike back. Ira Gifford summed up Reverend Kynett's subversive activities in a letter to Annie Wittenmyer on August 16th:

> Mr. Kynett has ignored all connection with the aid societies that you represent and set upon his own hand employing agents in the field, Reverend Truesdale and one other Reverend, and is acting very foolish and obstinate in many ways. And in this he has gone so far as to make complaints to the Governor "saying that he was not counseled at the time my appointment was made and that he has

> been pushed aside, etc." All untrue, and the best of it is that he meets with no special favor from the Governor, but rather, put the Governor on inquiring. Which will work to his disadvantage in the end. So I pay but little attention to his whining. Merely ask of him for the sake of our suffering soldiers not to do anything that will prevent their getting at this time what they very much need.[307]

Reverend Kynett's assertion that he had not had a hand in Ira Gifford's appointment is untrue. The minutes of the meeting reported in the *Davenport Daily Gazette* in May underscored that Reverend Kynett had interceded on Ira Gifford's behalf and had been instrumental to the appointment. However, Reverend Kynett had obviously become less than pleased by Ira Gifford's decision to support Annie Wittenmyer, which was likely the true cause of his change of heart.

Ira Gifford concluded that Reverend Kynett had repudiated the agreement to cooperate. Instead, Reverend Kynett had proceeded under his own authority to try a build a parallel organization to distribute goods and provide reports from the front that his organization needed to compete with Ira Gifford and Annie Wittenmyer's activities. His Machiavellian strategy of setting up a shadow structure appeared to be alienating the good graces of the governor, according to Ira Gifford.

That September, the actions of the Iowa Legislature and governor confounded Reverend Kynett's attempts to dominate soldiers' relief and marginalize Annie Wittenmyer, Ira Gifford, and Archibald. Governor Kirkwood called a special session on September 3, 1862, to address "some questions vitally affecting the public welfare" that required immediate attention.[308] For the governor, sanitary affairs were the first question of vital importance for the special session. Governor Kirkwood announced that, "The provision made for our sick and wounded soldiers, and for their return to their homes on furlough, will under existing circumstances prove wholly inadequate. The largely increased number of our soldiers that will shortly be in the field, and the great length of time they will be exposed to the danger of disease and the casualties of battle, will render absolutely necessary a large increase of the fund provided for their care and comfort."[309]

Archibald, Ira Gifford, and Annie Wittenmyer knew that the governor intended to have legislation introduced at the special session related to expanding sanitary relief to the soldiers. Prior to the start of session on August 27th, Archibald penned a short but revealing missive to Annie Wittenmyer, imploring her to go to Des Moines to lobby for the relief aid. Archibald mentioned that he wrote Colonel Ira Gifford about the sanitary affairs matters and that the two of them had discussed what they thought needed to be done. Archibald said in his letter to Annie Wittenmyer that he was "convinced that [Annie Wittenmyer] should return to Iowa and represent matters there during the sitting of the legislature in a proper light [and] be the clarion of the cause in which we are laboring to unite."[310] Annie Wittenmyer did go and she lobbied to profound effect.

In addition to an increase in the funding, the legislature and governor appointed Annie Wittenmyer as state sanitary agent by statute. The legislature adopted Chapter 36, An Act to provide for the appointment of Sanitary Agents and to define their duties.[311] Section 1 of the Act authorized and required the governor "to appoint two or more agents (one of whom shall be Mrs. Annie Wittenmyer) as Sanitary Agents for the state of Iowa."[312] While Annie Wittenmyer immediately was appointed, Governor Kirkwood later used the authority under this statute to appoint Archibald. Reverend Kynett, however, was not appointed under this legislative grant of authority.

The legislature and governor intended to elevate Annie Wittenmyer to the new office of State Sanitary Agent. The effect was to give her official state powers. It put her at least on par with Reverend Kynett. Perhaps it was meant to resolve the rivalry in her favor. It may have also been the governor's way of putting Reverend Kynett in his place.

Archibald found out about Annie Wittenmyer's success at the legislature session in a letter from her, dated September 15, 1862, that she penned from Des Moines, Iowa. She wrote to Archibald for help. She needed him to get her a pass in order to return to the front.

On September 25th, Archibald responded with his own letter. He had read Annie Wittenmyer's letter "with great pleasure and hastened to comply with her very reasonable request" for an order of passage from John G. T. Holston, medical director for the District of West Tennessee and Corinth. Archibald passed along Mr. Holston's gratification that she had been successful at the Iowa Legislature session in "procuring the passage of [her] favorite measures for the relief of the sick and wounded soldiers and that [she] was honored by [the Iowa Legislature] with a position [Iowa state sanitary agent]."

The elevation of Archibald from contract surgeon of the 13th Infantry to first assistant to John G. T. Holston, medical director for the District of Western Tennessee and Corinth, happened like many things in war—very quickly. Much had happened at the front after Annie Wittenmyer left to lobby the Iowa Legislature at the special session in early September.

In early September 1862, a Confederate Army under General Sterling Price approached Corinth from the east along the Memphis and Charleston Railroad line. To the south of Corinth, another Confederate Army under General Van Dorn approached. These maneuvers were a continuation of the probing strategy the Confederate forces had tried with skirmishes at Bolivar, Tennessee, that Archibald had witnessed in late August. General Grant could not afford to let these forces converge. He could not let them slip past him into Western Tennessee.

General Grant gathered troops and resolved to confront Confederate General Price's army before General Van Dorn could join General Price or come to his aid.[313] General Grant had the Union troops around Bolivar, including the Iowa 13th Infantry Regiment with Archibald, brought by railroad to Corinth. By consolidating his troops, he had a mobile army of 9,000 in addition to the garrison at Corinth.

On September 18th, General Grant planned to attack General Price on two sides at Iuka with troops led by General Rosecrans and General Ord. The Iowa 13th Infantry Regiment was with General Ord. General Rosecrans ran into stiff Confederate resistance and suffered heavy casualties on September 19th, although he was ultimately successful in causing the Confederates under General Price to retreat from Iuka.[314] The Union troops under Rosecrans suffered over 700 casualties.

The Battle of Iuka was the prelude to a later, second battle for Corinth, which was the bigger prize. Iuka, Mississippi, lay along the railroad east of Corinth. It apparently was not very large. Ira Gifford described it as a "forlorn desert, called by courtesy a village."[315]

After the battle, Colonel Ira Gifford brought soldiers' relief aid down to the wounded soldiers. He met Archibald and learned of his promotion. Colonel Ira Gifford passed along news of Archibald's latest honor, explaining that Archibald "was taken from Corinth to assist the medical director at Iuka; there he labored with his accustomed energy and kindness, and so effectively as to receive the highest endorsements from all connected with the army at that point."[316]

In the aftermath of the battle, Archibald rose to become the first assistant to John G. T. Holston, the medical director for the District of Western Tennessee and Corinth.[317] Archibald served in an administrative capacity as surgeon inspector general on General Grant's medical staff during this time.[318]

In this position, Archibald received high praise for his medical service. The medical director himself penned a letter of recommendation to Governor Kirkwood on September 21st recommending "Dr. Maxwell of your state to your most favorable notice and assure you that any medical commission bestowed upon him, no matter how high the trust, would be a trust safely reposed."[319] The surgeon for the Iowa 11th Infantry Regiment also wrote a letter of recommendation, stating that he "had been watching Dr. Maxwell most closely in his intercourse with the soldiers both as a general superintendent to look after this interest and a physician" and found him "well fit for any capacity he may be put in."[320]

While Archibald was focusing on treating the wounded, Colonel Ira Gifford and Annie Wittenmyer continued the work of bringing forward the greatly needed relief aid from Iowa for the soldiers.[321] The contending armies had created a vast food desert. Colonel Ira Gifford remarked that the "surrounding region had been stripped of edibles and forage that nothing could be obtained for the wounded or for troops after the fight [at Iuka] until supplies were taken from Corinth."[322]

Archibald was not able to stay in his new position very long after the Battle of Iuka. Family obligations called him to return to Davenport, Iowa. Very soon after his return, he was offered an opportunity to continue rendering service to the Union cause without leaving Iowa.

CHAPTER 13:
To Keokuk Goes a Professor and an Assistant Surgeon

In October 1862, Archibald returned to Iowa, to begin a new chapter in his war service. He received two different appointments in Keokuk, Iowa: an appointment in the military hospital and one at the college in Keokuk. In the years after the war, Archibald looked back on this period with the fondest of affections.[323]

While Keokuk, Iowa, today is a small, river town, Keokuk during the Civil War was a medical center and busy river port. The College of Physicians and Surgeons had established itself in Keokuk in 1850. The state legislature of Iowa recognized it as the Medical Department for the State University. Early in the war, an army medical hospital was located within the medical school in 1861. In late April 1862, the hospital expanded to include other buildings like the Estes House in order to accommodate the increasing number of wounded Union soldiers flowing north up the Mississippi from the battle of Shiloh on the river steamer *D. A. January*.[324] In August 1862, the hospital consisted of four buildings: the Estes House, the medical college, the Leighton House, and the Public School House, with the Estes House as the central point for distribution of supplies.[325] Both the Estes House and Leighton House were hotels that the army converted to use as hospitals. By October 1862, the Keokuk Army General Hospital had expanded yet again, from four buildings to five.[326]

On October 18, 1862, the Army Surgeon General's Office appointed Archibald assistant surgeon of volunteers under Surgeon of Volunteers M. K. Taylor at Keokuk Army General Hospital in Keokuk, Iowa.[327] While his formal appointment, as shown in the picture of the appointment letter, did not come through until October 18th, Archibald was already on the job at Keokuk on October 16th.[328]

The College of Physicians and Surgeons in Keokuk also offered Archibald a professorial chair position.[329] He happily accepted it and taught Physiology and Pathology. The position dovetailed well with his other appointment in Keokuk. The

College faculty taught in sessions 16 weeks long and began in October. At the beginning of the session in October, he described the attendance as "unexpectedly large for war-times." [330] The high attendance may have been in response to a greater need for trained doctors.

Archibald's decision to accept the offers in Keokuk did not make everyone happy. The editor of the *Davenport Daily Gazette* expressed his opinion in the October 18th newspaper that he "sincerely hoped that [Archibald's] services may be secured in some position where his skill can be employed for the benefit of our sick and wounded soldiers, and therefore trust he will decline the proffered professorship."[331]

The newspaper was not the only source of pressure on Archibald to decline the positions in Keokuk. Ira Gifford and Annie Wittenmyer considered him for an appointment in the new organization that Annie Wittenmyer was setting up after her September appointment as state sanitary agent. In an October 6, 1862, letter, Ira Gifford proposed that the governor appoint Archibald to inspect hospitals for Annie Wittenmyer's new organization.[332] Ira Gifford must also have written of the possibility to Archibald.

Archibald wrote Ira Gifford a letter on October 16th stating that he declined at that time to take the positions offered by Ira Gifford and others, including any position in the field with Annie Wittenmyer's new organization, the Iowa Sanitary Commission. Archibald said, that he had "met the Governor who offered [him] a Surgeonship of a Region, General Sanitary Agent or any other appointment that [he] could name in that connection."[333] He had declined any such appointment, explaining, he "had been appointed Professor of Physiology and General Pathology of the Medical College of [the state of Iowa]" located in Keokuk.[334] He also was busy as an Assistant Surgeon "with a charge of a Division" at the Keokuk Hospital.[335] Archibald left the door open to consider future appointments, writing, "I thought to hold off until I could see in which capacity I could do the most good."[336] Ira Gifford subsequently circulated the letter to Annie Wittenmyer. As a result, she set aside for a time pressuring Archibald to accept an appointment.

Archibald had many reasons unstated in his letter for declining appointments in the field in October 1862 and accepting the teaching professorial position at the medical college. The appointment to the professorship represented the pinnacle recognition of his professional expertise in the medical field. The same drive for excellence and recognition that pushed the fatherless farm boy to get an education and a profession made turning down such an opportunity difficult. He also likely accepted because it fit with the high value that he placed on education in general; prior to the war he had served on the Davenport School Board.

While these factors may have played a part, family obligation was likely a key reason for his decision to stick closer to Davenport. Archibald needed to be near Davenport to treat and nurse his brother-in-law, John Cook Jr., back to health.[337] John, along with his Ohio regiment, had been with Union General Don Carlos Buell's Army of the Ohio chasing down Confederate General Bragg's army, which had slipped into Kentucky. Because John had some medical training, his regiment assigned him to take care of the wounded in Lebanon, Kentucky. There, he had fallen gravely ill with a lung ailment, likely tuberculosis. The army furloughed him so that he could return home to recover or die. John did not return to Ohio, but instead travelled to Davenport, Iowa, in October 1862. Under Archibald's supervision, his family nursed John back to health at Archibald's home in Davenport. Eventually John recovered and finished his medical schooling in Keokuk where Archibald taught.

Additionally, Archibald's financial condition was not stable. He had volunteered early in 1862. While the governor had paid him $311.62 for his time after Shiloh, he had been in search of an appointment with pay. The opportunities in Keokuk as a professor and with the Keokuk Army General Hospital represented an opportunity for a regular source of income. Income must have been sorely needed in the face of a long summer, which saw the foreclosure of a number of his investment real estate properties.

Finally, Archibald believed that he was doing his duty to the cause. He closed his October 16th letter to Ira Gifford stating that he "had attended the election and voted to suppress rebellion—save the Union and support universal freedom. To do so, I used a ballot."[338] Archibald's remark in the context of the letter reminded Ira Gifford that there were many ways to support their aims. Archibald's reference to a ballot contrasts with the unstated other "b" word—bullets—which Union soldiers were using to advance the same cause. Both were needed; and both were important. Also, it was an ever-important reminder that Archibald believed strongly in the system of democratic government.

Two days after his letter, Archibald was officially appointed as Assistant Surgeon of Volunteers reporting to M. K. Taylor, Surgeon and Head of the Keokuk Army General Hospital. Dr. M. K. Taylor placed Archibald in charge of the 8th Street Hospital, which had been a Keokuk public school house until it was converted to use as a hospital.[339] The hospital was a basic brick schoolhouse divided into two wards.[340] As the surgeon in charge of the hospital, Archibald was responsible for several hundred patients.

Within days of his arrival, Archibald had an impact in an unexpected corner—halting loan sharking practices exploiting Union soldiers. On Wednesday, October 29, 1862, the *Davenport Daily Gazette* published his letter that brought to light the exploitation of wounded, furloughed Union soldiers, which he referred to as a "sharp game."[341] It was a common practice to furlough wounded soldiers so that they could return home to recover from their illness and wounds or die. The furloughed soldiers often were low on cash or penniless, because the paymaster had not forwarded their pay. Archibald noticed that loan sharks were advancing furloughed soldiers' money at 20%, 40%, and 50% interest, which he described as "[shaving] their papers (demands on government)."[342]

His letter brought the practice to the attention of the public and Governor Kirkwood. Four days later on Saturday, November 1st the *Davenport Daily Gazette* reported that Governor Kirkwood had "appointed J. C. Todd, Esq. [of Davenport] as a State Agent to proceed to Keokuk" to open an office to lend money at no interest to the soldiers on furlough.[343] The furloughed soldiers used the money to travel home or for immediate needs on furlough. Mr. Todd then coordinated with the army paymaster in St. Louis to collect sums due the soldier. The amount advanced was deducted from the pay and the rest of the pay forwarded to the soldier.

In addition to halting exploitation of the soldiers, Archibald continued to earn high praise for his medical treatment of his patients. Ira Gifford inspected the hospital at Keokuk with Archibald on his way south to Rolla, Missouri, in November 1862, and praised Archibald's work. [344] In December, the local *Davenport Daily Gazette* reported that in private letters home, soldiers in Keokuk Hospital praised Archibald's attention and skill.[345]

Archibald and the other surgeons took part in a plan in late 1862 to consolidate and more efficiently operate the Keokuk hospital. By December 19th, the medical staff, including Archibald, had decided to consolidate the hospital into three buildings. The retrofitted hotels (Leighton House and Estes House) continued to serve as hospitals. In addition, the government rented a new facility, the Simmons House. As part of the consolidation, Archibald and the other medical staff moved over 1,800 patients out of the medical college, 8th Street, and 4th Street facilities, which was more patients than the whole hospital had in August.

While Archibald was busy laboring in Keokuk, Reverend Kynett was busy trying to thwart Annie Wittenmyer. Ira Gifford bore the bad news in an October letter to Annie Wittenmyer. Ira Gifford informed Annie Wittenmyer that Reverend Kynett and his supporters attempted to undermine her through reports they sent to the governor that were critical of her and her methods. Reverend Kynett's attacks on Annie Wittenmyer were severe enough that Reverend Ingalls of the Iowa 3rd Cavalry rose to defend her in a letter published in the *Davenport Daily Gazette* on December 13, 1862. [346] While Reverend Ingalls in his letter does not name the "critics" casting ungenerous criticism of Annie Wittenmyer, it appears evident from Ira Gifford's letter to Annie Wittenmyer that Reverend Kynett and his supporters were the source of the criticism and "aspersions" in the newspapers.

Reverend Ingalls characterized the critics' reports as "failing to reach an intelligent comprehension of hospital wants," because the reports were based on interviews that resembled "calls of etiquette in city society, when [the troops] were in barracks which were easy of access by the best modes of travel."[347] These "visits" to Reverend Ingalls "looked like nice recreation, or trips of sightseeing and pleasure."[348] The critics made "inquiries of Colonels, Surgeons, and Chaplains, to secure" data from which to make their deficient reports because they did not visit the hospitals and speak with the common soldiers.[349] In short, Reverend Ingalls believed that Reverend Kynett and his supporters were not interested in getting their hands dirty and had no clue what the real soldiers' relief needs were.

When these reports began to appear, Ira Gifford raised the issue when he visited Governor Kirkwood. Governor Kirkwood said that he "had little confidence in the reports coming from Kynett and did not rely in the least upon the statements made by Truesdale," who was an agent of Reverend Kynett.[350] Ira Gifford was happy to relay that quote to Annie Wittenmyer. It suggests that the Reverend Kynett was not convincing the governor, but the governor may not have been the primary intended audience. Instead, the audience may have been the supporters of Reverend Kynett in the state of Iowa.

In contrast to Reverend Kynett's group, the governor was pleased with Annie Wittenmyer. Not only the governor was pleased, but Reverend Ingalls in his letter also had high praise for her, stating that she had "evinced the greatest assiduity and care in faithfully performing her duties" as Iowa state sanitary agent and her selection was "fortunate for both the benevolent at home and the suffering soldiers in the field."[351] According to Reverend Ingalls, Annie Wittenmyer knew better the needs of the soldiers because she and members of her organization had experience treating the common soldiers. As he put it, Annie Wittenmyer had engaged in "careful inspection of the camps in their sanitary condition, speaking to each soldier in the hospital tent, and to the sick scattered through the quarters; inquiring their wants and wishes, addressing in the name of the ladies of Iowa, words of comfort to the pale and emaciated, and often representing mother and sister by the side of the dying soldier."[352]

This raises an interesting question: If the governor was so disappointed with Reverend Kynett and his group, why did the governor continue to tolerate him? The governor may have thought that the two organizations together yielded more donations than one organization by itself. Moreover, Ira Gifford, Archibald, Annie Wittenmyer, and others were concerned that Reverend Kynett might do something that would "embarrass" the sanitary affairs movement. An embarrassing incident or political infighting might affect the free will donations required to meet the needs of the soldiers. Also, Reverend Kynett had political supporters. There may have been a real fear that if the governor took action to remove Reverend Kynett, it might turn into a scandal, which could damage the soldiers' relief effort and could reduce desperately needed donations. As Annie Wittenmyer's star rose, Reverend Kynett's political supporters demonstrated a long reach and a more than passing talent for political gamesmanship.

At the October meeting with Ira Gifford, Governor Kirkwood previewed some upcoming appointments. The governor had already spoken with Archibald and understood that at least for the time being, Archibald was content to labor in Keokuk. Instead, the governor intended to appoint John Clark and Dr. Ennis "to cooperate with [Annie Wittenmyer]."[353] Governor Kirkwood "persuaded Ira Gifford "to go once more into the field, instructing Clark and Ennis to report to [Ira Gifford]" in Davenport. Mr. Clark was to replace Ira Gifford, who was not able to continue.[354] Dr. Ennis was to fulfill Archibald's intended role providing medical aid to Iowa soldiers and inspecting medical facilities.

While both Dr. Ennis and Mr. Clark went with Ira Gifford on his last trip in November 1862 to bring supplies down to Helena, Arkansas, and into Mississippi, Dr. Ennis and John Clark were not enduring appointments. Dr. Ennis was not in good health. Mr. Clark resigned when illness struck his family. Within four or five months, both Mr. Clark and Dr. Ennis resigned, leaving a hole in Annie Wittenmyer's organization that she approached Archibald to fill.

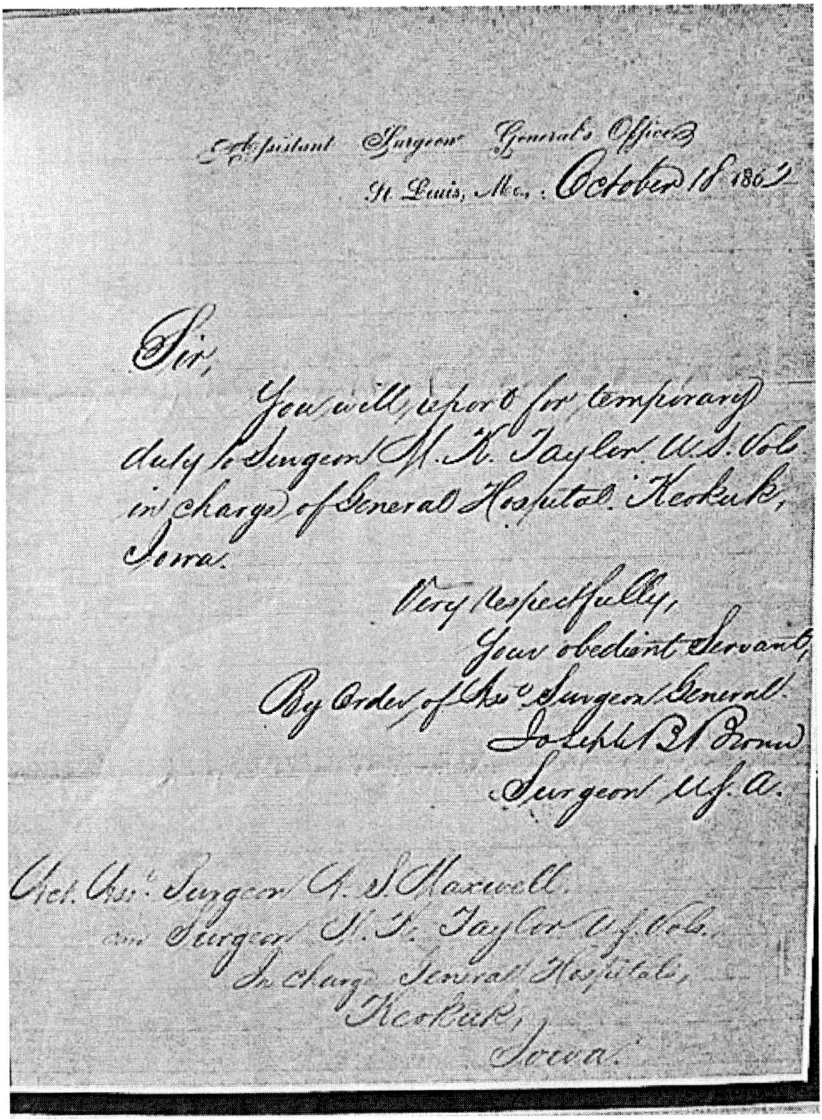

Assistant Surgeon General's Office
St. Louis, Mo., October 18 1862

Sir,

You will report for temporary duty to Surgeon M. K. Taylor U.S. Vol. in charge of General Hospital Keokuk, Iowa.

Very Respectfully,
Your obedient Servant,
By Order of Asst. Surgeon General
Joseph B. Brown
Surgeon U.S.A.

Act. Asst. Surgeon A. S. Maxwell
on Surgeon M. K. Taylor U.S. Vol.
In charge General Hospital,
Keokuk,
Iowa.

Letter appointing Dr. Archibald S. Maxwell as assistant surgeon of volunteers in Keokuk, Iowa. Picture reprinted with permission and courtesy of Mary Christenson.

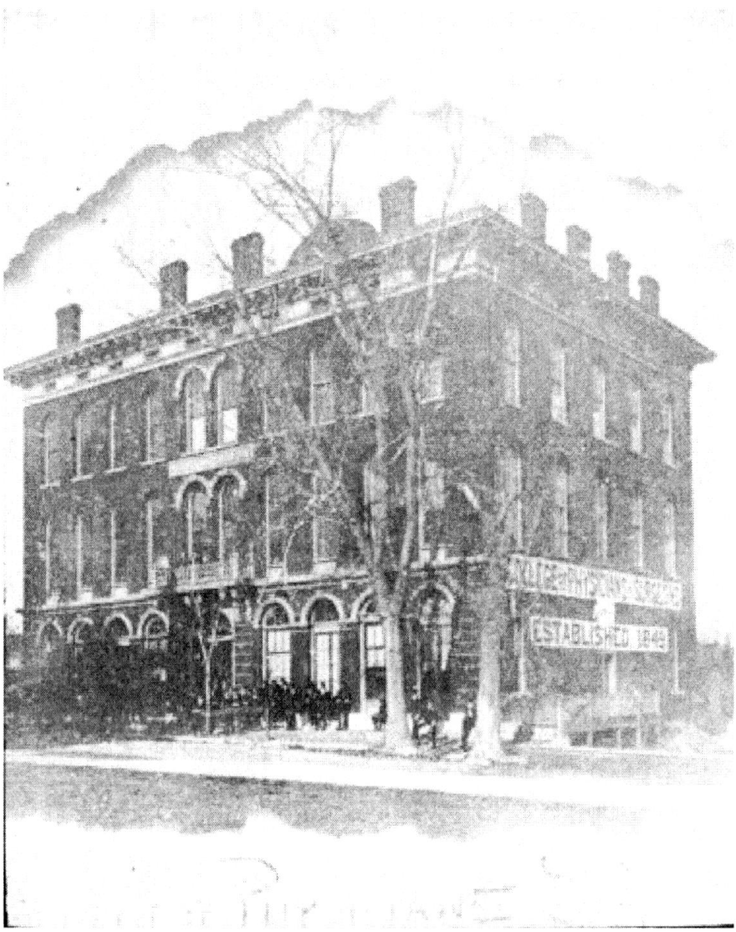

Photo of College of Physicians and Surgeons, Keokuk, Iowa, 1860 provided courtesy of the University of Iowa.

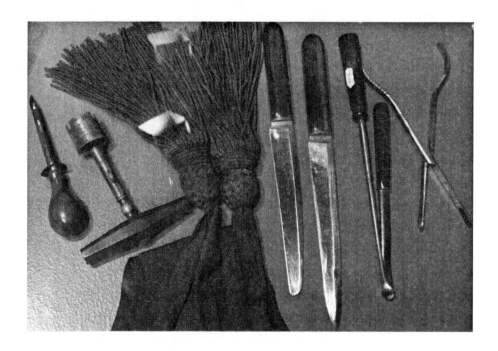

This is the author's picture of Archibald's civil war surgery kit, which is on display at the Putnam Museum in Davenport, Iowa. Author took the picture with the permission of the Putnam Museum. The tools from left to right are as follows: (1) a sharp trocar for draining cysts; (2) a cylindrical trephine saw for drilling a hole in the skull to relieve swelling in the brain; (3) two amputation knives; (4) a spoon like bullet scoop; (5) a flattened steel elevator for removing bone during trepanning; and (6) a bullet forceps for removing a projectile. The medical kit was donated by George A. Maxwell, who was the author's grandfather. Archibald also had a bone saw, which is not pictured.

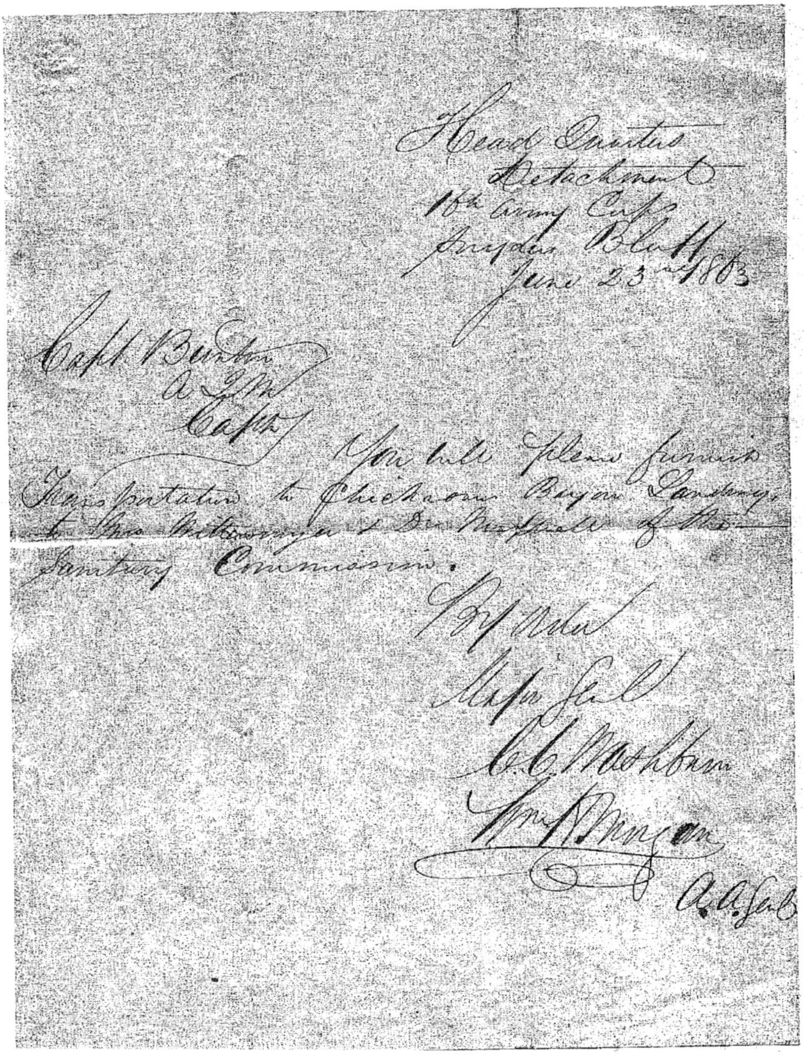

Head Quarters
Detachment
16th Army Corps
Snyders Bluff
June 23rd 1863

Capt. V Burton
A Q M
Capt.

You will please furnish Transportation to Chickasaw Bayou Landing to Mrs Wittenmyer & Dr Mitchell of the Sanitary Commission.

By Order
Major Genl
C C Washburn
Wm H Morgan
A A Genl

June 23, 1863, transport order for Archibald and Annie Wittenmyer.

CHAPTER 14:
To Vicksburg and Back

With the resignations of John Clark and Dr. Ennis, Annie Wittenmyer decided in the spring of 1863 to persuade Archibald to return. Annie Wittenmyer wanted Archibald's assistance in providing soldiers relief in connection with the campaign to take Vicksburg and Port Hudson, which was in full motion. She wrote him a letter probably in late March 1863 to inquire about his willingness and availability to rejoin the service and help her out.

Annie Wittenmyer was concerned about the increasing amount of sickness in hospitals in Helena, Arkansas, and other points along the Mississippi. Her circulars published in the early part of the year underline this growing problem, which was a natural result of the change in strategy for taking Vicksburg and Port Hudson. [355]

General Grant's original plan had been to proceed down along the Central Mississippi Railroad to take Vicksburg, using the railroad as the conduit for moving supplies to support the army. At the end of 1862, General Grant suffered a temporary setback when his supply depot at Holly Springs, Mississippi, was captured and destroyed by Confederate raiders.

After the loss of supplies at Holly Springs, General Grant changed course and moved down the Mississippi to secure dry ground on the east side of the river from which Union soldiers could threaten Vicksburg. The Union Army spent much of early 1863 moving down the river. This effort concentrated wounded along the Mississippi River.

In 1862 after major battles like Shiloh and Fort Donelson, the wounded had been loaded on steamers and sent to hospitals in the North. General Grant and other generals noticed that this policy deprived them of the pool of lightly wounded soldiers who, once recovered, could be sent back into the fight.[356] In the Vicksburg campaign, the army changed the protocol, which necessitated the establishment of hospitals nearer to the front with sufficient capacity and supplies to meet the wounded's needs.[357] The new protocol led to complaints that the army violated Congressional law by failing to transfer back to their home states severely wounded soldiers who had been in hospital for three months.[358]

As part of this new protocol, military hospitals were expanded in Memphis, Tennessee, at the direction of Assistant Surgeon General Wood in early 1863. The military took over the "largest and best buildings in the city, having been originally designed for hotels or blocks of stores, four and five stories high. The hospitals were named Overton, Washington, Gayoso, Jackson, Jefferson, Marine, Webster, Union, Gangrene, and Officers and were capable of accommodating about 5,000 sick and wounded men."[359] The Union wounded from General Grant's successful campaign against Vicksburg filled the hospitals in the summer of 1863, creating a constant demand for sanitary stores.[360]

While the workload increased, the two state sanitary affairs organizations appeared at odds with each other. By spring 1863, Reverend Kynett's Iowa State Army Sanitary Commission did not appear to be cooperating well with Annie Wittenmyer and her organization. Instead of jointly publishing sanitary circulars requesting donations, the organizations published competing circulars in newspapers throughout the state, sometimes in the same edition of the newspaper. The two organizations requested the same items but with different addresses for shipment of the goods. For instance, on March 14, 1863, Annie Wittenmyer's Iowa Sanitary Commission circular requesting that donations be sent to Partridge and Co. in St. Louis ran in the *Burlington Weekly Hawk-Eye*. Her circular had a note of support from Governor Kirkwood.[361] The same circular ran in the *Cedar Falls Gazette* the day before.[362] Less than two weeks later, Reverend Kynett's Iowa Army Sanitary Commission ran a similar circular on page six of the *Burlington Weekly Hawk-Eye* directing people to only send their donations to Davenport, Iowa.[363] These dueling sanitary circulars evidenced the continuing rivalry between the organizations.

The criticism of the sanitary affairs and soldiers' relief movement and of the lack of unity in the movement continued. Annie Wittenmyer addressed the criticism of her and the Iowa State Sanitary Affairs in a circular published on June 13, 1863, in the *Burlington Weekly Hawk-Eye*. She expressed "a desire to establish and maintain direct communication with every society in the State organized for the benefit of soldiers," which was a call to unity given the needs of the soldiers in the Vicksburg campaign.[364] She also recognized that "there will always be those who find fault, whose charity consists mainly in criticizing other peoples' labors," and drove the point home that efforts harmful to sanitary affairs hurt the troops.[365] Annie Wittenmyer appealed to "the wives, mothers, and sisters of our brave men now exposed to privations of camp life," and asked these women to "remember that those who discourage and embarrass sanitary efforts are the soldiers' worst enemies."[366]

In addition to publishing circulars to increase donations, Annie Wittenmyer began making other preparations to meet the needs of the Vicksburg campaign in March–April, 1863. She contacted Archibald, writing a letter that he called "interesting." While the text of Annie Wittenmyer's "interesting letter" does not survive, Archibald's April 12th response makes it evident that she asked if he would assist her as a state sanitary agent in the field. He responded to her question, saying that he was "willing to do almost any and every thing that proves to relieve the suffering soldiers," which signaled to Annie Wittenmyer to move ahead.[367]

While Archibald was interested, he had some personal affairs to "fix up" in Davenport before he could go. Archibald explained that he was no longer an assistant surgeon at the Keokuk General Hospital. Archibald had left the service and returned to Davenport, "owning to the unsettled condition of [his] business."[368] Even though he had resigned his commission in the army, he was still teaching at the medical college in Keokuk. He, in fact, explained that he intended to "return to Keokuk to lecture" later in April.

Archibald's April letter also passed along the latest and curious news about Annie Wittenmyer's rival—Reverend A. J. Kynett. Archibald noted that Reverend Kynett had been very sick but was recovering. Archibald said in his letter that he had "called once to see [Reverend Kynett]. [Reverend Kynett] had treated me kindly."[369] Archibald also added as an almost non sequitur that Reverend Kynett "owns considerable property." Archibald may have relayed these discordant statements to Annie Wittenmyer because it was of general interest to her.

Archibald also took the time to put in a good word for his eldest son, John, who would have been almost 15 years old. Archibald noted that, "my son is very anxious to accompany you. He has a high opinion of you and is preparing himself. He writes a better hand than your present clerk, and I guess would please you in other respects."[370] Annie Wittenmyer declined to hire a nearly 15 year old and instead retained a college graduate, Mary Shelton of Mount Pleasant.[371] This was not to be the last time that Archibald attempted to push forward the interests of his eldest son.

Meanwhile, General Grant and his Union Army on April 30th crossed to the east side of the Mississippi and captured Grand Gulf below Vicksburg, and then proceeded to move ever closer to Vicksburg. In early May, they fought and defeated the Confederates at the Battles of Port Gibson, Champion's Hill, and the Big Black River. By the end of May, General Grant and his army had driven the Confederate field army back behind the siege works at Vicksburg.

Annie Wittenmyer wrote to Archibald again in May, informing him of her efforts to get approval from the governor to have Archibald join her.[372] While the Union Army had suffered casualties in the battles and from the hard marching, Annie Wittenmyer knew that more casualties were coming from the assault on the siege works at Vicksburg. The Union Army assaulted the Vicksburg works on the 19th and 22nd and sustained heavy losses, which increased the urgency to deliver soldiers' aid and other sanitary supplies.[373]

At the time General Grant ordered his troops to make the opening assaults on the works at Vicksburg, Archibald wrote to Mrs. Wittenmyer the following:

> Dear Madam— Your very kind letter was received on yesterday. I thank you for the interest you manifest on my behalf. If you succeed, please have provisions made for funds ... for my departure as soon as I can get my private business arranged. Had I not better visit Dubuque, Iowa, before leaving South? Say to Gov. that Dr. Ennis could take Col. L.'s place at Keokuk and also act as Surgeon of the Border Rifle Regiment. If the Gov. does not appoint him, perhaps he would Dr. Saunders; [Dr. Ennis] told me he would accept [the governor], [Dr. Ennis'] health is much better. The little folk are all in State and all send you their best wishes. Nothing new here in Sanitary matter since you left. Excuse haste. Your most obedient servant. AS Maxwell. Please accept my photograph. ASM.[374]

Archibald's short letter of reply on May 20, 1863, conveys a sense of urgency in the language and sentence structure. He and, no doubt, Annie Wittenmyer, felt the urgency to gather and move the supplies down to the wounded at Vicksburg and its surrounding hospitals. However, Annie Wittenmyer was still working on securing his appointment. At the same time, Archibald's response is intensely personal. Despite the urgency, Archibald was clear that he wanted "funds" for his trip, which is in contrast to his prior trips in 1862. Given his business and other financial reverses in 1862, Archibald probably was not in a position to head off on a new endeavor without a source of income.

Annie Wittenmyer's shorthand on the side of the letter notes that four days later, she replied on May 24th, which demonstrated her sense of urgency to start the trip. In that timeframe, Annie Wittenmyer must have gotten permission for Archibald to travel in June in some capacity as an acting state sanitary agent. Whatever his capacity, he was not officially sworn in and appointed as state sanitary agent until August. Based on Archibald's correspondence, she instructed him to gather in one large sweep all the soldiers' relief and sanitary affairs supplies that could be found on his way down the Mississippi River to meet her.[375]

In his next letter written to Annie Wittenmyer on June 8th from Cairo, Illinois, on the steamer *Imperial*, Archibald chronicled his efforts over the prior six days to push the Iowa Sanitary Affairs' supplies downriver to Vicksburg.[376] He left Davenport on June 2nd, having made arrangements with a committee in Davenport to forward supplies as fast as possible. He then stopped in Keokuk for a day to make arrangements related to his professorship and other personal affairs, while at the same time ordering all supplies shipped downriver on the "first through boat" and "urging upon people to be liberal and keep sending at Keokuk."[377] After Keokuk, he stopped at Hannibal, where he found and shipped additional goods before heading to St. Louis. At St. Louis, he checked in with the Iowa Sanitary Commission's local representative, where he found his transportation order. Archibald confirmed that Annie Wittenmyer's office had already sent six tons of relief supplies south to Vicksburg, and that they would continue to ship them as more supplies arrived from Hannibal and Keokuk.

He arrived in Cairo on the *Imperial* at 8:00 a.m. on June 8th. Archibald had stopped there to gather additional supplies. Reverend Kynett's organization had also sent supplies ahead to a U.S. Sanitary Commission office in Cairo. Archibald had been told to bring those supplies as well. When he visited the U.S. Sanitary Commission's office looking for supplies that Reverend Kynett had sent earmarked for Iowa soldiers, Archibald wrote that he "found but few goods and was told" Reverend Kynett had sent none. Archibald suspected that something was wrong and visited the "principals [U.S. Sanitary Commission Agents] houses and found goods with Kynett's name on [them]."[378] Archibald learned that the Chicago Section of the U.S. Sanitary Commission had repackaged 50 boxes, 75 barrels and 2 kegs from Reverend Kynett's organization, and that these goods had been there four days or more and were being used by soldiers there. Archibald informed Reverend Kynett of the situation, but he had to keep moving.

Archibald's report on the loss of goods from Kynett's organization must have confirmed Annie Wittenmyer's main objections to how the U.S. Sanitary

Commission ran its operations. By commingling goods from different locations, Reverend Kynett and his organization effectively lost control of those goods and could not ensure that the Iowa wounded men received the benefit of them. The U.S. Sanitary Commission philosophically sought to commingle the goods and provide support where needed, regardless the source of the aid and the Union soldiers' home state. This was a philosophical difference in how to deliver the aid that continued to persist.

After Cairo, Archibald journeyed downriver and met up with Annie Wittenmyer. He brought to Vicksburg all the sanitary supplies that he could sweep up on his way. While he was there, Annie Wittenmyer and Archibald moved about the Union camps administering aid to the soldiers. Closer to the end of the siege on June 23, 1863, they procured a transport order to cross together from Snyder Bluff to Chickasaw Bayou Landing.[379]

When Annie Wittenmyer arrived at Vicksburg, she requested an ambulance, but the army gave instead a "fine silver mounted, easy carriage captured at Jackson." She and others of the team, which probably included Archibald, used the carriage to visit the field hospitals. Confederate sharpshooters in Vicksburg "sent more than a hundred shots after that carriage, supposing some high official was the occupant."[380] The shots fell low, chipping the wheels. After the fall of Vicksburg, a Confederate captain told Archibald about it. Archibald left the captain in shock when he informed him that the occupant was Annie Wittenmyer.

Archibald and Annie Wittenmyer endured more than just the sharpshooter bullets in administering the aid. Many of the field hospitals at Vicksburg had to be set up within range of Confederate siege guns, because a relieving army of Confederates under General Johnson was near, forcing General Grant to draw his lines in close.[381]

The closeness of the hospitals to the front lines created tough conditions for Mrs. Annie Wittenmyer, Archibald, and other members of her group. At the field hospital, Annie Wittenmyer later recalled, "The ceaseless roar of artillery, and scream of shot and shell; the sharp whirr of small shot just over our heads; the June sun blazing down upon us with torrid heat, and no shelter for the sick but the white canvas tents perched on the sides of the bluffs in places excavated for them, the bank cutting off the circulation of air,—were almost unbearable."[382]

Iowa State officials continued to visit the front lines as they had done after the Battle at Fort Donelson and on other occasions. Governor Kirkwood and other officials visited during the active siege at Vicksburg. While Governor Kirkwood met with Archibald in Vicksburg, Annie Wittenmyer does not mention Archibald among the group of "distinguished visitors" on their inspection tour of the siege lines. While he was there, Governor Kirkwood reviewed the sanitary efforts of his agents in the field to address accusations that the agents were misapplying goods entrusted to them. He found those accusations unfounded.

Finally, Confederate General Pemberton accepted General Grant's terms of surrender for Vicksburg. On July 4, 1863, Archibald and Annie Wittenmyer rose early and "drove out to General Logan's headquarters whence the army was to begin their triumphant march into the city."[383] Archibald and the ladies took their position on the battlements of Fort Hill, where they had a full view of the city. Annie Wittenmyer described the contrasting scene from that hill where before "the roar of battle had raged again and again about the fort, but now all was calm and still as the dawning of this day of peace. As far as we could see, the muskets were stacked, and white handkerchiefs were fluttering above them. The Confederate and Union soldiers stood along the lines in groups, talking as friendly as though they had never exchanged shot with intent to kill."[384]

She and Archibald stood and surveyed this hopeful scene. Annie Wittenmyer then explained, "As last the still was broken by the tramp of horsemen; General Grant with his staff of officers following passed near us and honored us with a military salute ... We stood there with our field glasses in our hands, watching them as they marched down into the city. There was a long halt. They approached each other forming into long double columns, and then we saw, opposite the blue, the gray forming into lines. There was movement forward of officers, the flash in the bright sunlight of swords as they were handed over to the conquerors, and then handed back."[385]

With the fall of Vicksburg, Annie Wittenmyer and Archibald entered the city as well. Annie Wittenmyer and her group entered on July 5th to inspect the Confederate hospitals and arrange to provide aid to the Confederate wounded there. Annie Wittenmyer had arranged for Mr. Yeatman of the Western Sanitary Commission in St. Louis to send her supplies "in anticipation of the surrender, for the Confederate hospital in Vicksburg."[386] As Annie Wittenmyer described, "the hospitals were in the most wretched condition; the men being without beds or pillows or any other comforts for the sick."[387] Given the extent of the siege and exhaustion of supplies, it is not surprising to learn that the hospitals were in the condition that she found them.

Annie Wittenmyer and her group, including Archibald, planned to use Vicksburg as a base of operations. General Grant assigned Annie Wittenmyer and her team a large house in town to use as headquarters, and she lived there along with Archibald and the wife of General Stone.[388]

By the end of July 1863, Archibald and Annie Wittenmyer needed more donations. Annie Wittenmyer returned to Iowa in late July to gather more supplies and ensure the final arrangements for Archibald's formal appointment as Iowa state sanitary agent by the governor. To get the word out on the type and kind donations needed, she had their joint circular published in the Iowa newspapers signed by Annie Wittenmyer and Archibald as Iowa state sanitary agents. Archibald and Annie Wittenmyer explained that "the number of the sick has been largely increased by excessive labor, loss of sleep and hardships during the siege of Vicksburg."[389] They also informed the Iowa people that their wounded would not likely to be shipped north, which increased the need for sanitary supplies. They requested "shirts, drawers, towels and rags" as well as various fresh and canned vegetable and fruit stores be sent to Mrs. Annie Wittenmyer care of Partridge & Co. in St. Louis, Missouri.[390]

Annie Wittenmyer and Archibald's request for vegetables and fruits coincided with similar requests by the regional Western Sanitary Commission and the U.S. Sanitary Commission. Early in the spring 1863 campaign for Vicksburg, the Union soldiers' health had begun to show signs of scurvy due to improper diet.[391] The Western Sanitary Commission and the U.S. Sanitary Commission made efforts to address and prevent scurvy with a steady supply of vegetables.[392] Even in July and early August, Archibald and Annie Wittenmyer continued to combat scurvy in the troops with requests for fruit and vegetables.

Annie Wittenmyer made clear to Archibald that she wanted his assistance as state sanitary agent. She had Archibald's name added to the *Sanitary Circular* with his new title, State Sanitary Agent, even though he had not formally received it. [393] While time must have been pressing, Mrs. Annie Wittenmyer obviously saw value in having Archibald's name on the circular along with hers.

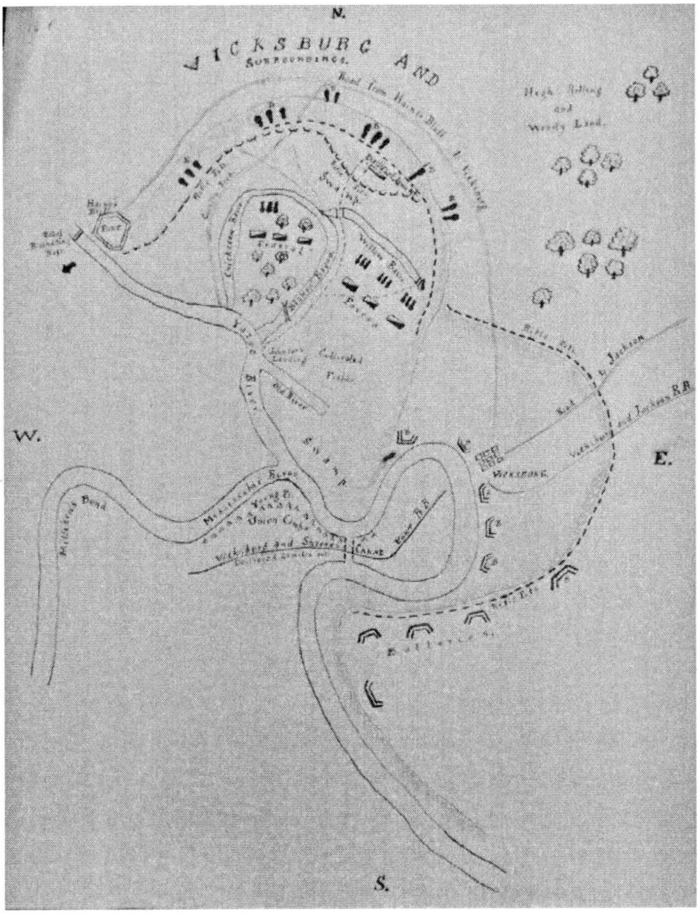

Map of Vicksburg Siege Lines found in Archibald's correspondence to the governor. Courtesy of the State Historical Society of Iowa.[394]

CHAPTER 15: The Last Run Down the River—Hospital Inspections and the End Game

In St. Louis on August 4, 1863, while on his return trip to Iowa, Archibald picked up a short letter from Annie Wittenmyer that welcomed him with the news of his upcoming appointment.[395] In her August 3rd letter, she said, "Your appointment is confirmed—I have seen the Governor—he will appoint you—wishes you to come up to Iowa City when you return."[396]

While the news of his appointment was welcome, Annie Wittenmyer made clear that Archibald's appointment was due to her request. She had lobbied Governor Kirkwood. Archibald had only "to come up to Iowa City" when he returned to Iowa to be confirmed. Given the governor's past support for Archibald, it appears strange that Archibald needed that much assistance. It also confirms the power Annie Wittenmyer had in Iowa sanitary affairs. Finally, it is possible that Annie Wittenmyer's intervention was necessary because Governor Kirkwood had a lot to wrap up before embarking on his new diplomatic appointment in Denmark.

In the same August 3rd letter, she confided to Archibald her concerns that Reverend A. J. Kynett was up to his old tricks again. She wrote, "Everything favorable in the State except Mr. Kynett's continued attempts to embarrass Sanitary Matters."[397] She promised to give Archibald "further details when I see you."[398]

Mrs. Annie Wittenmyer likely referred to Reverend A. J. Kynett's efforts in August 1863 to expand the Iowa Army State Sanitary Commission's network at the expense of Annie Wittenmyer's network in northeast Iowa. Reverend Kynett recorded in his final report that in August 1863, the Iowa Army State Sanitary Commission had taken steps to expand "in the Northern part of the State."[399] Reverend Kynett had enlisted two women from the Ladies Aid Society of Dubuque to "supervise the work west and north of Dubuque."[400]

In response to this new development, Annie Wittenmyer dispatched Archibald on his only official state tour as state sanitary agent to address an immediate threat to her network in Dubuque and towns in Northeast Iowa. On August 19, 1863, Archibald reached West Union, which is located about 81 miles north and west of Dubuque in northeastern Iowa. In a letter to Annie Wittenmyer that day, he updated her on his efforts to thwart this new threat from Reverend Kynett's organization. Archibald wrote, "I have progressed this far on my tour, having visited all points on the review up to Dubuque, from there the several villages to Decorah, and then from there to this place and have been fortunate in enlisting the interest of the people in our great enterprise."[401] Archibald made clear that he viewed the tour as successful from Mrs. Annie Wittenmyer's perspective, reporting, "I think I have somewhat interfered with Rev. Kynett's arrangements."[402]

On the tour, Archibald visited camps and gatherings designed to collect donations to be distributed to the wounded and sick soldiers. After leaving West Union, he was to go west and southwest to attend "a camp meeting."[403] The proceeds from refreshments sold at the camp meeting would go to the local ladies aid society. Archibald planned to "meet and speak with citizens and society" there on August 20th. [404] He then planned to continue heading south and east and arrive back in Davenport around August 30th.

While it might be possible that Annie Wittenmyer sent Archibald on the tour of Northeast Iowa to assist in Reverend Kynett's efforts to establish his donation network, it seems unlikely. Annie Wittenmyer was justly proud of her network's ability to collect goods and did not welcome inroads. She wrote with great pride to Governor Kirkwood on December 18, 1863, "From all the information, I can gather, I have received since serving the last fifteen months, five-sixths of all the goods coming from the State."[405] Based on her estimate, Reverend Kynett's organization only collected one-sixth. In this light, Archibald's tour was to ensure that Annie Wittenmyer's network continued to receive its share of the goods and to frustrate Reverend Kynett's new strategy to gather donations of supplies from Northeast Iowa.

Having explained his efforts on behalf of the Iowa Sanitary Affairs office, Archibald asked for a huge favor from Annie Wittenmyer: assist Archibald in setting his eldest son John up with a business opportunity in the newly conquered South. Archibald knew he was asking a big favor, because the wind-up began with "now my kind friend." Archibald explained, "I have an offer to get my son in business provided I can get a permit to sell goods in Vicksburg or some other good point on the river. Will you please make the requisite inquiry of Major General Grant, and if he will grant such a permit upon any condition, then please procure it in favor of John H. Maxwell and [Company] in this [company] you can of course be one if desirable. If this cannot be procured, could you learn the chances at Helena and Memphis and you quietly oblige me?"[406]

While Archibald used the term company, he was proposing a partnership with his son, John H., as the named visible partner and other silent partners. John H. Maxwell was 15 years old, which was a bit young to run a business selling goods in a newly pacified area of the South without parental assistance. However, given the politics of the time, it may have caused a scandal for a state sanitary agent to be openly operating a for-profit concern that relied on vital connections gained through his or her position as state sanitary agent.

Annie Wittenmyer replied to him that, "I want no business chances" and need not "speak to Grant."[407] This was the politically and legally wise thing for her to do. In fact, Archibald's request was unwise, and he should have known better given Reverend Emond's allegations against Annie Wittenmyer circulating at time.

In early 1863, Reverend Emond of Iowa City had accused Annie Wittenmyer of selling the sanitary goods rather than distributing the supplies. Annie Wittenmyer did not need to add any fuel by appearing to abuse her position for personal financial gain. The accusations made against Annie Wittenmyer by Reverend Emond in early 1863 did not fade away but continued to persist. In the July 30th *Sanitary Circular*, Governor Kirkwood had taken the accusations against Annie Wittenmyer head-on. He wrote, "Many accusations have been made against Annie Wittenmyer, and other Sanitary Agents, that they misapply the goods sent them, and that the soldiers fail to receive [the supplies.] I have recently visited the army, and had ample opportunity to learn the merits of Annie Wittenmyer's work, and I am fully satisfied all such charges against her are utterly false."[408]

In this light, his offer to Mrs. Annie Wittenmyer to be a silent partner in the enterprise could have been incredibly damaging to her. While the business Archibald proposed was completely separate from the distribution of sanitary goods and supplies to the soldiers, it had the ability to be twisted and seen as an improper abuse of her position for personal financial gain. Also, although the accusations of Reverend Edmond were unfounded, such allegations might have gained currency if she was known to be participating in a for-profit enterprise in Union-held parts of the South on the basis of permits obtained using her friendship with General Grant. After all, if it had been safe for her to be a known partner in the business, there would be no reason to offer her a "silent" partnership in John H. Maxwell and Company.

Archibald presumably let the matter rest when he returned to Davenport to begin for his next trip down South to inspect hospitals in late 1863. John H. Maxwell did accompany his father on that trip, but it does not appear that he engaged in business. While Archibald's business proposition strikes us today as potentially crossing ethical and legal boundaries, the boundaries on such matters were less clear in Archibald's day.

When back in Davenport at the end of August, Archibald arranged to gather sanitary supplies to bring with him. To spur donations, Annie Wittenmyer had another letter published in Iowa newspapers discussing the great need of the wounded and sick at Helena, Arkansas.

Sometime in September, Archibald left Davenport and headed south. He stopped at St. Louis and at Cairo to pick up additional supplies. On the evening of October 7, 1863, he arrived in Memphis, Tennessee, with "over 200 tons of sanitary goods" on the *Clara Belle* steamer.[409] His trip down the Mississippi to that point had been "extremely tedious" and risky due to the low stage of the water.[410]

Unlike previous trips when Archibald visited large concentrations of troops along the Mississippi, Archibald instead stopped in many places and ranged quite far to find the Iowa regiments and soldiers who were the objects of his medical care and assistance. After the fall of Vicksburg, the main theater of the battle in the west shifted to Chattanooga, in Eastern Tennessee. However, the Union Army massed around Vicksburg was broken up, sending the Iowa regiments to multiple places. Some shifted east to Chattanooga. Some remained around Vicksburg. Others went south and west, pursuant to General Halleck's orders to secure Texas and Louisiana. The United States was particularly concerned that France or another European power might interfere by trying to grab part of Texas.[411]

At the time of Archibald's arrival in Memphis, Union General Sherman and his army prepared to cut their way through Confederate General Johnston's blocking force on their way to assist General Rosecrans.[412] The Union troops engaged in extended skirmishes trying to push through. These movements set the stage for the later battle at Chattanooga, Tennessee. At the time, Archibald decided to remain in Memphis with his medical and sanitary supplies, because he believed that a major battle was about to occur around Corinth, Mississippi, which would require his medical expertise and his supplies.[413]

While he waited, he went out to inspect the major Union hospitals in Memphis: Gayoso, Overton, Union, Webster, Jefferson, Adams, Washington, Jackson, Officer's, and Church. At these Memphis hospitals, Archibald began to collect statistics on the number of soldiers in the hospital with various diseases and the treatment administered, along with the number who returned to duty, the number who died, and the number still in hospital. He divided statistics on diarrhea into acute and chronic for each hospital. At Church Hospital, he also gathered statistics on gangrene and encephalitis. As he went farther south, he changed his list of diseases to include dysentery and "fever."

Archibald chose to study these serious diseases and the efficacy of various treatments to identify ineffective from effective treatments for these ailments. He expressed that he hoped by "presenting largely accumulating collections of the course of treatments most practiced in the Southwestern Armies with the results in the most dread diseases" to help other doctors improve their outcomes.[414] Archibald's study was similar to other efforts to identify more effective treatments by observation in the field. The army under Surgeon General Hammond and his successor Surgeon General Barnes compiled a book with new practices called the *Medical and Surgical History of the War of the Rebellion*. Army surgeons submitted samples of their reports. Also, army surgeons submitted their observations to journals such as the *American Medical Times*.

Archibald's study and statistics had several problems, which probably prevented him from making any particular recommendation. First, there was no set definition of diarrhea or dysentery, or any particular line between acute or chronic diarrhea.[415] For some surgeons, blood in the stool was an identifier of dysentery; but for others, it was not. Because of the lack of common definitions, there was an inherent likelihood of inconsistency as one surgeon's definition of dysentery differed from another. Moreover, the categories did not represent modern notions for diagnoses of dysentery and diarrhea. With regard to diarrhea acute or chronic, there likely was a range of things that may have caused it, from bad or ill-cooked food to any manner of virus or bacterial infection, but the limits of medicine in the Civil War did not permit investigation at that level.

As far as treatments went, doctors felt differently, as Archibald's own records attest, about how to treat such diseases. Some doctors believed bad diet to be linked to diarrhea. Of those that blamed diet, some thought it due to ill-prepared food, and others thought it due to the typical soldier's diet of beans, pork, and hard tack. A third group believed it to be due to an absence of fresh food. As his constant calls for better food make plain, Archibald believed that diet was key and thought food preparation, typical army diet, and lack of fresh food all played a role. To a certain extent, he was probably right.

This is not to say that Archibald's statistics are not potentially useful. They provide a window into the health and recovery of the Iowa soldiers in the Mississippi area after the fall of Vicksburg. They also provide information on the vast array of treatments, including a number of substances used as medicine that are today known to be lethal and of no, or limited, medical value.

In addition to statistics on dysentery and diarrhea, Archibald also noted some additional diseases prevalent at that geographic location at the time. In Memphis, Archibald recorded statistics for gangrene at Church Hospital, where the surgeon was using a pioneering bromine acid treatment to kill hospital gangrene. This treatment involved injecting bromine acid into the gangrene wound with a syringe and topical application of a weak bromine solution on the wound.[416] Archibald likely observed this treatment being done by associates of Doctor Goldsmith, the Superintendent of Hospitals in Louisville, Kentucky. Surgeon Goldsmith had developed and published the medical procedure in early 1863.[417]

Having collected the data, Archibald used it in his written report to support his conclusions about the medical facilities that he inspected, although his final, published report omitted the statistics for unexplained reasons. In the early part of the trip, Archibald was not pleased with conditions and care in the Memphis hospitals. He reported to Annie Wittenmyer in a letter on October 19, 1863, in terse sentences. "Hospitals are in but fair condition. . .Those hospitals are not what they should be. Recoveries are not rapid nor certain."[418] While Archibald does not explicitly state it, he likely compared the Memphis hospitals' practices and conditions with those in the Keokuk General Hospital where he had recently served in hospital. Implicitly, he found the hospitals in Memphis not up to the Keokuk standard.

By looking at the statistics from the Memphis hospitals, it is possible to see what dismayed Archibald about treatment and recoveries. The vast majority of soldiers with cases of diarrhea either died or remained in hospital over the month-and-a-half period (September and half of October) that he was there. A very low percentage of the soldiers returned to duty. When compared against other hospitals in Archibald's survey, the Memphis hospitals' numbers were comparatively worse.[419]

Archibald stayed with the Iowa troops out of Memphis as they advanced east across Tennessee to La Grange, Tennessee. He followed the Iowa regiments inspecting the conditions of 2nd, 4th, 5th, 19th, 10th, 17th, 25th, 26th, 30th, and 31st Iowa infantry regiments, as well as the 1st Iowa battery. He supplied the regiments with much-needed vegetables and other sanitary supplies. On October 19th, he wrote to Annie Wittenmyer that "I have closed my visits to Tennessee on this line of communication" having inspected the regiments there, which he reported to be in "fair condition." His original reason to delay in Memphis—the likelihood of a big battle—did not materialize.

Archibald left Memphis on Sunday evening of October 25th in a steamboat bound for Vicksburg. He arrived in Vicksburg at noon on October 28th. When he arrived, he had the misfortune to learn that General McPherson had given Annie Wittenmyer's house to someone else, a Mrs. Simmons. The new occupant had given a number of the sanitary stores left there by Archibald and Annie Wittenmyer to the Soldiers Home that was established outside Vicksburg on August 6th. When Archibald called on General McPherson to discuss this change of affairs, General McPherson had "coolly remarked that if there was a house vacant that would suit her, that he would get [Annie Wittenmyer] one when here."[420] Because Archibald was only in town for a short period of time, he did not care about the house, but he was worried about the stores that had been given away.

Archibald immediately visited the Soldiers' Home and the sanitary depots to check on the level of supplies. He reported to Annie Wittenmyer the oft-repeated request for "vegetables." At the supply depots, he met Mr. Plattsburg, the Western Sanitary Commission agent in Vicksburg. While Archibald had yet to see it himself, the people on ground assured him that the health of the army regiments in the immediate Vicksburg area was "good or improving."[421] Unlike Reverend Kynett and his agents who had a reputation for relying entirely on such summary statements, Archibald did not intend to settle for such a cursory review. He visited the Soldiers' Home where soldiers could rest and grab a meal, reporting that 250 soldiers took supper.

After his initial visits to the sanitary depot and Soldiers' Home, he then set out to inspect McPherson Hospital and Confederate hospitals 1, 2, and 3 in Vicksburg on October 30th. The Hospitals that Archibald referred to as "Confederate hospitals 1, 2, and 3" were the hospitals that the Union Army had taken over when the city fell to them on July 4, 1863. He and Annie Wittenmyer had a particular connection with hospitals because Annie Wittenmyer's organization and the Western Sanitary Commission had arranged to provide medical supplies for those hospitals the day after the Union captured the city.[422]

After inspecting the hospitals and seeing to his affairs in Vicksburg, he visited on November 1, 1863, a group of troops two miles south of Vicksburg that formed Crocker's Iowa Brigade: the 11th, 13th, 15th and 16th Iowa Infantry Regiments. The Iowa Brigade was a veteran, disciplined formation that had fought together since Shiloh and were known for swift marches. At this camp, he found the "health of the troops improving." However, Archibald once again noted in his report that "vegetables needed very much." Archibald found the 11th and 13th Regiments in fairly good shape, with between 70–75% of their reported strength active for duty. Their rates for diarrhea and dysentery for September–October ranged between 9–15%, with a return to duty rate of 60–70%. However, even within the same camp, Archibald found startling differences. The soldiers in the 15th and 16th Iowa Infantry Regiments had a higher total of diarrhea and dysentery infections, and they had a lower rate of recovery and return to duty.

In his request for better and more nutritious food, Archibald made special note of the Iowa Brigade's heavy marching in August, September, and October 1863. In those three months, Crocker's Iowa Brigade had been north of Vicksburg, then conducted a month-long expedition in Louisiana, and then marched east of Vicksburg, and finally stopped at their camp two miles south of Vicksburg, where Archibald found them. Archibald reported that despite the heavy travel, their sanitary condition was good. However, their tents were "very poor." He recommended that the old ones be "turned over and new ones drawn."[423]

After visiting the regiments two miles south of Vicksburg, Archibald set out to visit the 2nd Iowa Battery at the Big Black River Bridge, which is about 20 miles east of Vicksburg. The battery's strength was at 60%. Archibald recorded diarrhea and dysentery rates for the September and October period of 38% and 37% of the effective force, respectively, which meant that, together, over half of the force had been sick with diarrhea and dysentery during that period at one point.[424] Nearly all recovered and returned to duty, but illness was at a staggeringly high level and no doubt cut into force effectiveness.

Once he had concluded his inspection of the 2nd Battery, Archibald travelled back towards Vicksburg until he reached the camp of the 3rd Brigade and the 4th Iowa Cavalry. This force had pitched camp nine miles east of Vicksburg at Clear Creek. The 3rd Brigade consisted of the 8th, 12th, and 35th Iowa Infantry Regiments. At the time of his visit, Archibald found that two of the infantry regiments in the 3rd Brigade were at close to 50% strength. The Colonel for the 8th infantry informed Archibald that in August, the brigade had camped on Big Black River and gotten an illness described as a fever. The 3rd Brigade had moved a mile west in search of a better location, which they had believed would improve their health. Despite its weakened state, the 3rd Brigade had joined in an expedition near the capital of Mississippi, Jackson, in September. When the expedition had ended, the brigade and the cavalry regiment had returned to its present location at Clear Creek.

The fever that the detachment had picked up in August at Big Black River burned through the three infantry regiments in the 3rd Brigade and the 4th Cavalry regiment, during the September–October 1863 time frame. [425] This fighting force had a total of 1,900 effectives out of a nominal strength of over 2,400. Out of those 1,900 effectives, a total of 993 soldiers got sick with fever, or nearly 50% of the effective force. Archibald provided little context to the "fever" during that period, but it likely was the same infection, given that it passed through the entire brigade and cavalry regiment during the same September–October timeframe. Archibald felt that diet played a part in the brigade's illness. He authorized "fresh bread, potatoes, onions, fresh beef (two days a week) . . . with sanitary supplies for the sick and convalescent."[426] In recovering from the fever, the 8th and 12th Infantry Regiments had a high rate of soldiers return to duty, with few deaths.

The medical condition of the 12th and 8th Infantry was in deep contrast to the third regiment in the brigade, the 35th Infantry. Under the onslaught of the fever, its soldiers did not fare well, with over half of their fever victims still in hospital at the time of Archibald's report. Archibald pointed the finger at the 35th Infantry's surgeon in his report, writing, "The 35th Infantry from the want of an experienced surgeon has suffered much and now is the same as destitute."[427] Despite blaming principally the surgeon, he expressed the opinion that the medical problems of the 35th represented deeper-seated, structural medical issues and required the Iowa Legislature to consider "procuring medical surgical aid."[428] Archibald also failed to point out the 4th Cavalry was in not much better shape, as 110 of its 353 were still in the hospital.

Despite the problems with the 35th Infantry Regiment, Archibald found the troops around Vicksburg generally in good shape. During that time, he examined "the quarters, fixtures, and hospitals" of all the regiments and found most of them to be "in very excellent condition."[429] He reported that in a span of five days from November 1st to November 5th, he had visited all the commands. He also assisted in tracking down missing records, like the death certificate for a soldier that passed in a hospital in St. Louis, Missouri.

He did add his usual lament that the "sanitary goods are most poorly given out by distributing agents."[430] Archibald had complained about distribution problems since Corinth in May of 1862. His observation suggests that the sanitary commissions continued to stumble in the final step of distribution to the actual soldier, despite the considerable improvements in gathering the donations and moving the goods down their logistical supply chain to a forward depot. Accordingly, it explains why he constantly ferried supplies out to the soldiers on his visits.

After that last lament, he closed his report covering Vicksburg and Memphis and prepared to board the steamer in Vicksburg bound for New Orleans on November 7, 1863. On November 9th, he stopped at Natchez, Mississippi, and received a brief report on the Iowa 3rd Infantry Regiment -there, but could not stop, as he had with him 176 Iowa soldiers returning from furlough to their regiments in Southern Louisiana. On November 11, 1863, he arrived in New Orleans.

He went to Union General Bank's headquarters, where he obtained orders to facilitate his travel about Louisiana.[431] He learned the locations of the Iowa regiments scattered throughout Louisiana, with some on their way to Texas by boat.

While in New Orleans, Archibald toured and inspected the United States General Hospital's five buildings and convalescent camps. Archibald explained that his inspection was not the cursory pass through or just "calling on the men," but instead, "learning by all means, the attentions needed and whether [the wounded] received them."[432] Once again, he highlighted the general method used by Annie Wittenmyer and him, which contrasted with the higher level and less-investigative inspections done by Reverend Kynett's organization.

In his inspection of the hospitals, Archibald found some practices he liked and other practices that he did not. He praised the New Orleans army hospitals, finding that they had been "provided with almost all the modern appliances of the best hospitals and mostly conducted on the most vigorous system of hygiene notions."[433] The surgeons and officers were "gentlemanly in their attentions;" he thought they had good bedside manner.

As a whole, he noted that the surgeons' use of medication "is mostly *judicious*", although not held in "very high esteem" by some of the surgeons.[434] He singled out St. James Hospital as the only hospital where surgeons treated patients with medication by their diagnosis, or as he referred to it "attention to classification of cases for medication." In contrast, Archibald found surgeons in other hospitals in New Orleans that prescribed in some cases no particular plan of treatment for individuals suffering from diarrhea.

Archibald lodged his usual complaint that the food for the sick and wounded did not meet his standards. The New Orleans hospitals suffered from "a great lack in all of the cooking arrangements and diet." He stressed that "the food does not reach the *patient* in a *condition* that is fit for *sick men*."

To be specific, his complaint was that the food was not prepared and served in a manner to be consumed by sick men. Archibald was satisfied with the type and variety of the food due to the "magnificent hospital fund" that provided the means for the hospitals to be "supplied with everything the market affords." Earlier in the war, Archibald made a similar observation when the army tried to feed its sick and wounded on marching rations with no utensils after the battle of Fort Donelson. Ever since, Archibald made a habit of taking notice of such bad practices and rooting them out. In New Orleans, he brought the issue to the medical officers in charge, and they promised a change.[435] Annie Wittenmyer took this a step further later in the war with her special kitchens that she ran through the Christian Sanitary Affairs Commission.

In his inspection of New Orleans hospitals, Archibald found the 13th Army Corps Hospital to be a squalid, cold nightmare of a place filled with bad food and worse doctors. The army had converted a former cotton press into a hospital. The hospital was in an old, two-story shed structure built in the form of a hollow square open in the front. The converted building did not provide good ventilation or hold in warmth, which in November–December was important. Archibald found the doctors there used poor judgment in prescribing medication, hygiene was neglected, and the food defective.[436] Archibald reported the terrible circumstances to the medical director and expressed his medical opinion that the patients there needed to be moved to other hospitals. The medical director promised, "to correct the evil."[437]

In addition to inspections, Archibald also practiced medicine. After inspecting the 13th Army Corps Hospital, he went out to two nearby convalescent camps and, during the inspection, prescribed a highly unusual treatment for individuals suffering from chronic diarrhea and dysentery. He suggested to the doctor-in-charge that these suffering soldiers ride horses through mounted infantry evolutions for several hours each day.[438] Archibald thought it would be beneficial, although to modern sensibilities that type of treatment seems unconventional and unlikely to assist in recovery from chronic diarrhea. His prescribed treatment was emblematic of this era of medicine, which grasped at solutions without understanding the underlying bacterial and viral causes of many infections. His prescribed treatment of exercise was likely less dangerous than some of the substances given as medicine, although that is probably all that can be said for it.

After wrapping up his inspections in New Orleans, Archibald left to see the regiments outside the city. He ordered and brought along vegetables and other sanitary supplies for the Iowa troops stationed outside the city that he intended to visit. He also placed orders and arranged to ship supplies to Iowa troops that he was not able to see for one reason or another, such as the 1st Iowa Battery, which was camped at Brasher City in Berwick Bay.

Leaving New Orleans, Archibald journeyed 180 miles north and west to visit the 24th and 28th Iowa Infantry Regiments at New Iberia, Louisiana. The troops skirmished and mopped up rebel resistance in the area. Archibald found the troops in New Iberia in better physical health and shape than they had been on July 1st during the Siege of Vicksburg. Archibald attributed the health to the abundant food available in the New Iberia region, which had been appropriated by the Union troops.

Archibald was delighted that the 24th and 28th were in such good shape, because their medical hospital at Franklin, Louisiana, did not meet his standards. He called the General Hospital there "but an excuse" for a hospital. [439] Given the context, the hospital was likely a miserable place. He found the medical appliances "insufficient." He was thankful that only two Iowa soldiers were there at his inspection. Outside of noting it in his report, he does not mention having brought it to anyone's attention, which was uncharacteristic of Archibald. However, Archibald may have not had anyone in that remote locale that he could approach about it.

After his visit to New Iberia, he travelled to Algiers, Louisiana, to see Iowa Regiments, the 21st and 22nd, before they departed for Texas. By the time Archibald made it to Algiers, half of the 21st and 22nd Iowa Regiments had already shipped out for Texas. He regretted that he missed the first half of those regiments and "could not furnish them with any vegetables," which they would need in route.[440] He also missed the 19th, 20th, 34th and 38th Regiments because they had left for Texas before he arrived. He did not flinch from seeing that the troops received their vegetables and made arrangements to ship them vegetables in Texas.

Because he was in the area, the governor and Adjutant General Baker requested that Archibald investigate the tragic deaths of many in the 38th Iowa Infantry Regiment. Archibald checked into the treatment of the sick from the 38th Regiment at various hospitals in Louisiana. He found that a great number of its men had fallen fill and not survived their service in Louisiana. During his trip, Archibald did "find many of the poor suffering members of that command and rendered them important relief" in the various hospitals along the way.[441] He also gathered the names of the deceased from hospitals along the river. He checked into a report that a great number of the soldiers in the 38th Regiment had died in Port Hudson and Baton Rouge hospitals, but the hospital records in those locations were so bad that he could not confirm the reports. He apologized that conclusive answers to their questions evaded him.

Before leaving New Orleans on December 4, 1863, Archibald procured the furlough and discharge of medical cases to enable the boys to go home. He advocated for the release of these soldiers with the medical director and got approval. Some of the furloughed men were sent home to Iowa via New York, which was deemed the "best route for the safety and health of the invalids."[442] Archibald and others determined that a ship around Florida and up the east coast was faster and better than a slow steamship ride up the Mississippi River against the river current.

On December 9th, Archibald finished his report in Vicksburg, Mississippi. On December 10th, he followed up with an additional report from Vicksburg on the changes in the health of the regiments at Vicksburg during the month that he had been in New Orleans. He found the Iowa Brigade had remained in the same camp location. Archibald was concerned. He observed that although "many are not sick", the character of the sickness was "very serious—displeasing—of a typhoid character."[443] He worried that the sickness might spread.

Having sent his last report, he left for Iowa. He planned to leave by the first boat for Memphis, and then from there to Cairo. He asked the governor or Adjutant General Baker to leave a telegraph for him in Cairo if they wanted him to journey to Chattanooga, Tennessee.[444] Annie Wittenmyer had already left for Chattanooga. Archibald did not receive a telegraph, so he returned to Iowa.

His war service was over, although he may not have known it at the time. Upon his return, Archibald submitted his report to Governor Kirkwood, who apparently was happy with it.[445]

While he had been busy in Vicksburg and New Orleans, momentous changes had occurred in Iowa Sanitary Affairs to change the nature of it for the rest of the war. These changes were caused by two separate, back-to-back sanitary affairs conventions in the fall of 1863. The first sanitary affairs convention in October 1863 was held in Muscatine, Iowa.

The second convention was called in Des Moines, and it began on November 18, 1863. Annie Wittenmyer's supporters in Keokuk asserted that the second was called "through hostility to Annie Wittenmyer, and the object is to kill her off by fair means or foul."[446] Annie Wittenmyer and her supporters mustered delegates to send to the second convention to prevent the opposition from pushing her out. Letters from a "Friend of the Soldier" published in the newspapers questioned the goals of the second convention as unrealistic solutions and provided strong arguments to support the current system. At the second convention in November, Mrs. Darwin gave an impassioned defense of female sanitary agents in the field, and Annie Wittenmyer in particular, to applause of many in attendance.[447]

The second convention in November led to the creation of a "permanent sanitary organization called the Iowa Sanitary Commission."[448] The new commission cooperated with both the U.S. Sanitary Commission and the Western Sanitary Commission. It spelled the end of Reverend Kynett—he submitted his final report, and the Iowa Army State Sanitary Commission closed. The second convention did not directly end Annie Wittenmyer's involvement, as she was appointed by the legislature. In fact, her supporters largely carried the day, although many of Reverend Kynett's supporters also were brought into the new organization.[449] She remained as the state sanitary agent for the time being and cooperated with the new commission.

The new united Iowa Sanitary Commission that emerged from the second November convention also took up the task of creating a Soldiers' Orphans Home for the orphans of Iowa's civil war soldiers. Annie Wittenmyer had publically championed the cause of this new institution to address a growing need. She and Archibald had conceived of the idea of a Soldiers' Orphans Home in Jackson, Tennessee in 1862.[450]

Having failed to prevail at the second November Convention, the adversaries of Annie Wittenmyer did not go quietly into that good night. In December, Reverend Norris of Dubuque gave a highly critical speech of Annie Wittenmyer's organization and the Western Sanitary Commission with which she worked.[451] Others continued their criticism in what some dubbed the War on Annie Wittenmyer.[452]

Archibald returned to this political stew from his trip inspecting hospitals in the South. While Archibald had been out, the controversy surrounding Annie Wittenmyer had gone from the slow boil of the summer to out of control. Although he may not have known it, more drama was in store when the 1864 legislative session convened.

In his parting 1864 State of the State Address, Governor Kirkwood praised the Sanitary Association's efforts to provide relief. Governor Kirkwood recommended that the state and the association continue to work together but that government leave day-to-day matters largely in the hands of the private associations. He also recommended continuing the practice of having a "liberal contingent fund" pay to assist and to "keep in the field such agents of the state as may be necessary."[453] This was his parting advice to the legislature and the recently elected Governor Stone.

Governor Kirkwood also submitted his summary of sanitary affairs expenses to account for funds appropriated in 1862. With regard to his sanitary agents, Governor Kirkwood believed they had all "done their duty faithfully" and had done much to aid Iowa soldiers. [454]Governor Kirkwood represented that Reverend Kynett's expenses and salary had been paid in full, but that Archibald and Annie Wittenmyer had unsettled accounts.[455] Governor Kirkwood expected Governor-elect Stone to pay any balances due. Shortly after Governor Kirkwood gave the speech, he left for his diplomatic appointment to Denmark.

The unpaid expenses left Archibald and Annie Wittenmyer vulnerable to objections to their unreimbursed expenses by the newly convening legislature. Through this crack, the enemies of Annie Wittenmyer forged a plan of attack. Their plan also allowed them to probe the unproven accusations that Annie Wittenmyer had sold sanitary supplies to Iowa soldiers.

Reverend Kynett may have known this tactic might be used. Reverend Kynett's pressured Governor Kirkwood to "draw on the balance due" and to pay his expenses promptly when Reverend Kynett submitted his report early on December 9, 1863.[456] Reverend Kynett did it a second time in a separate letter on December 29, 1863.[457]

Early in the session, Annie Wittenmyer submitted a long, comprehensive report to the Iowa Senate and House covering her term of service from its beginning up to that point, including a description of expenses.[458] She noted that the governor had appointed three sanitary agents to assist her in that time. The first two, Dr. Ennis and Mr. John Clark, were obliged to resign due to health issues after only a few months of service. She praised Archibald, who had replaced them starting in June. She reported that Archibald had "continued to labor with great ability and a zeal worthy of so good a cause up to the present time. His labors have extended over the greater part of the South-West and are spoken of with great commendation."[459]

After the initial reports, the enemies of Annie Wittenmyer unleashed their attack on February 6, 1864. The House standing committee on Sanitary Affairs passed a resolution calling the new Governor Stone to answer as quickly as possible several questions related to state sanitary agents appointed under the authority of September 1862 law. These state sanitary agents included Annie Wittenmyer, who was appointed by the law, and any additional state sanitary agents appointed by the governor under the authority granted him by the statute.[460] Because Reverend Kynett had not been appointed pursuant to that statutory authority, it very neatly avoided any questions directed at him. The resolution requested the following information:

(1) Which persons other than Annie Wittenmyer did Governor Kirkwood appoint using the authority provided by the legislature in the September 1862 law;

(2) What money, if any, did Governor Kirkwood provide to Mrs. Annie Wittenmyer and any other appointed Sanitary Agents under the September 1862 law, and how were such funds spent by the sanitary agents;

(3) "Whether the needed articles therewith purchased were furnished gratuitously to the sick and wounded soldiers in the field or whether said articles were sold to said soldiers, and if sold, what disposition was made of the proceeds of such sales;"

(4) What amounts were paid by Governor Kirkwood and then Governor Stone to Mrs. Annie Wittenmyer and the other agents as just and reasonable compensation, and what amounts were paid as travelling expenses; and

(5) Whether Annie Wittenmyer's travelling expenses associated with travelling to sanitary conventions and fairs were reimbursable expenses by the state.[461]

Because Annie Wittenmyer and Governor Kirkwood had already submitted reports providing a list of sanitary agents and an expense report, the House intended to dig deeper into the expenses to possibly find something that could be used to damage Annie Wittenmyer's reputation. While the question about whether Annie Wittenmyer had sold the articles was the heart and soul of the probe, the legislature clearly meant to see if there was anything to be made out of the salary and travel expenses as well. The legislature knew it was putting Governor Stone in a vise, because the events related to the questions had occurred under previous Governor Kirkwood administration.

In response, Governor Stone showed the fortitude necessary to reimburse Annie Wittenmyer what was due her, even after the controversy exploded. On February 10, 1864, four days after the House passed the resolution, he paid Annie Wittenmyer the $1,660.77 due her.[462] Given the circumstances, Governor Stone stood by Annie Wittenmyer even at the risk that his actions might worsen the crisis.

Governor Stone was less helpful in managing a response to the questions in the House's resolution. When he formally responded a week later on February 13, 1864, Governor Stone provided only evasive statements. While clearly Governor Kirkwood had left good records and Adjutant General Baker remained on staff, Governor Stone claimed partial or near total ignorance, stating that he "cannot be expected to give a history of the administrations of my predecessors, when they have left no records, " which was not true.[463] Nevertheless, Governor Stone had communicated with Governor Kirkwood, who informed him that Governor Kirkwood had appointed Dr. Ennis and Archibald. Archibald had served for nine months at $140 a month until the start of Governor Stone's administration. Governor Stone then deferred to Annie Wittenmyer's report to address the remainder of the questions from the Iowa House of Representatives before launching into how he wanted to reshape the sanitary affairs in his administration.

In her response to the resolution, Annie Wittenmyer, as she had done before, took the matter head-on, addressing each of the questions posed. Annie Wittenmyer defended her and Archibald's expenditures and salary. Archibald received $140 per month as compensation and $175 to cover expenses submitted to her.[464] She provided a detailed account of expenses with her report.

On the question related to the sale of sanitary supplies, Annie Wittenmyer defended herself with verve, explaining the circumstances that had given rise to allegation. During the Vicksburg campaign, few supplies were coming from the state, and Iowa regiments were desperately in need of sanitary supplies. In response to this great need, Annie Wittenmyer bought $300 in supplies with her own personal funds. With righteous indignation, she explained, "As I bought the supplies with my own money, and took them to the army at the risk of my life, and let them have them at *cost* and the *sick, without charge—there were no proceeds!*" (emphasis in the original).[465]

While not the clearest of responses, Annie Wittenmyer was saying that she had provided supplies at her own expense when supplies ran out during the siege of Vicksburg. She gave the supplies to the sick free of charge. Healthy soldiers in the Iowa regiments had also wanted access to the supplies that she had purchased. She consented but she required the healthy soldiers in Iowa regiments to purchase the supplies for the price that she had paid. She clearly was angry at the idea that one of her enemies had twisted her act of courageous generosity into an unfounded rumor that she was trying to profit from the soldiers' lack of supplies.

As for travel expenses to conventions and fairs, Annie Wittenmyer again defended Archibald by making clear that only she had attended conventions. She also destroyed the Iowa House members' objections by affirming that her attendance had cost the state of Iowa nothing. Yet again, Annie Wittenmyer left her enemies with little to grasp.

Archibald also felt compelled to defend himself, his expenses, and likely his friend Annie Wittenmyer as well. He submitted a letter to the House on February 18, 1864, which was referred to the Committee on Sanitary Affairs.[466] The Committee on Sanitary Affairs did not to publish his reply, because it probably did not add any new details. It must not have given them any more fuel for their investigation. His report also requested unpaid expenses of $55.92 related to his report.[467] The Iowa House of Representatives referred his expense request to the House Committee on Claims, who refused to pay the claim.

While the state repaid Annie Wittenmyer and Reverend Kynett their expenses, Archibald ended up footing the bill for the legislature's angst. Of the three, he was the one left with unpaid expenses. While $55.92 may not seem like much, the amount was more than one third of his monthly salary as a state sanitary agent.[468] Given that he had sacrificed and volunteered, he must have been disappointed to be denied repayment of expenses.

However, the members of the House were not done. The enemies of Annie Wittenmyer in the Iowa House continued to look for ways to fight back. While the members of the Iowa Senate passed resolutions in support of Annie Wittenmyer, House Member Vinton, in new legislation addressing sanitary agents and their compensation, attempted unsuccessfully to block women from serving as Iowa sanitary agents in the future.[469] While unsuccessful with his first try, House Member Vinton later in the session offered the following resolution:

> Resolved, that in the opinion of the members of the House of Representatives, the sum of seventy-five dollars per month, inclusive of all travelling and incidental expenses, is all that should be paid to each of the State Sanitary Agents employed under the provisions of

> the act approved on September 11, 1862, entitled "An Act to provide for the appointment of Sanitary Agents,"

The motion on the resolution carried 37 to 26.[470]

In one fell swoop, the House of Representatives opined that Archibald and Annie Wittenmyer had been overpaid for all their time and effort saving the lives of the legislators' brothers, neighbors, and relatives, and risking their own lives at the front. Because Reverend Kynett was not appointed under the Act, the Iowa House took no official stance of displeasure that Governor Kirkwood had paid Reverend Kynett $1,350.00 in salary and $405.50 in travelling and incidental expenses for a job that was performed mainly in Iowa. It also probably mattered little to them that at $75.00 inclusive of travel expenses, Annie Wittenmyer's proposed salary only barely covered her total travel expenses as State Agent of $1,097.58.

Archibald resigned in January 1864. His friend, Annie Wittenmyer, also resigned in April 1864 to pursue managing special kitchens for sick and wounded soldiers under the Christian Sanitary Commission.

This legislative drama likely upset Archibald, which may have effected how he chose to recall his service in the Civil War. When he retold the story of his service in later autobiographical summaries, he was circumspect about his service as an Iowa state sanitary agent. He stated that he "declined to accept an appointment from the governor as state sanitary agent or surgeon at large to operate in the field."[471] Archibald's statement is not true, based on the record. In his autobiographical snippet, he instead explained his role from June 1863 to January 1864 as the "sanitary inspector of hospitals," which is one thing that he did as an appointed state sanitary agent, but it was not the whole of his service.[472] He also claimed that the governor and legislature had given hearty approval to his service.[473] While the governor and many of the legislators no doubt were happy with his service, it is hard to characterize the legislative investigation and final resolution by Annie Wittenmyer's enemies as a nice gesture. His alteration of the record may have been his way to forget the manner in which he had been treated and his services devalued by the Iowa State Legislature.

Despite the ill-feeling caused by Annie Wittenmyer's enemies, Archibald remained justly proud of his service and sacrifice. At risk to his own life, he had answered the call of his fellow citizens to serve in his country's hour of need. He helped preserve the union and free the slaves. Archibald saved lives on the operating table, at the bedside, and by his efforts to improve hospital conditions and care for the sick and wounded soldiers.

After his resignation, he worked to publish his December 9, 1863, report to N. B. Baker, Adjutant General and Quartermaster on the hospitals in New Orleans and Louisiana in the Appendix of the *Report of the Adjutant General and Acting Quartermaster General of the State of Iowa January 1, 1863 to January 11, 1864*. The final published report does not include his earlier November 6, 1863 report, or the statistics that he gathered. Once Archibald and the Adjutant General Baker made the decision to exclude the statistics, the November 6, 1863, report may have required too many revisions to include in the final published work.

Upon his return to civilian life, Archibald settled back down in Davenport for the remainder of the war. He had a family to raise and a medical practice that beckoned him.

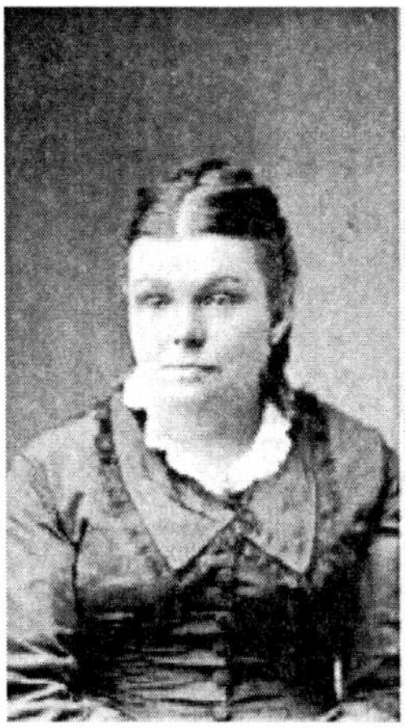 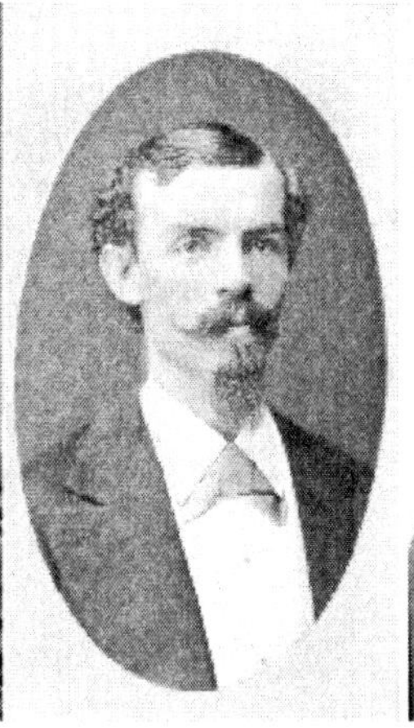 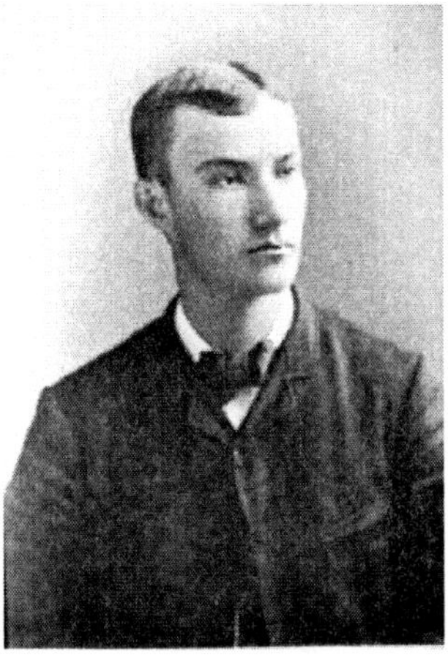

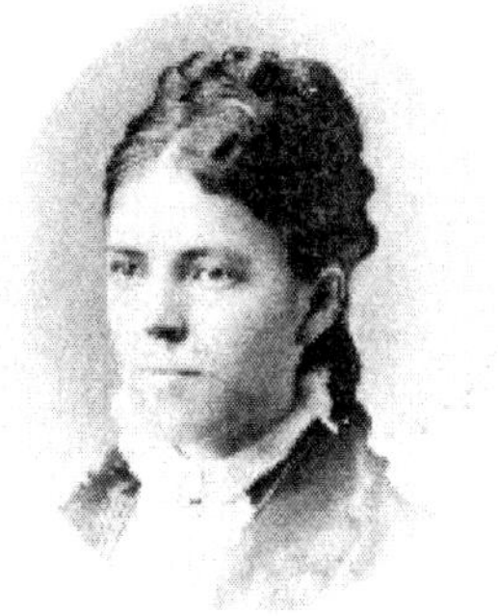 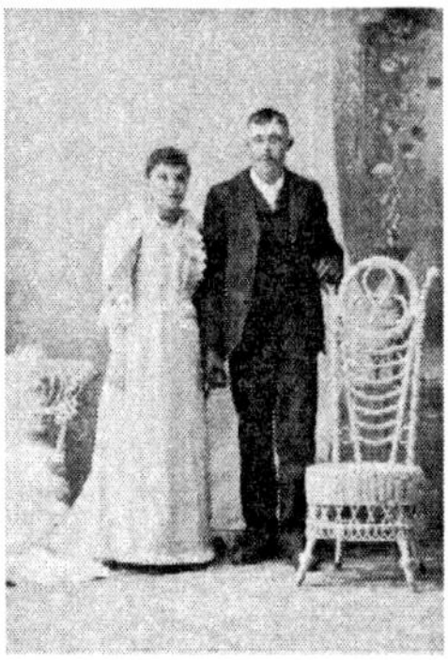 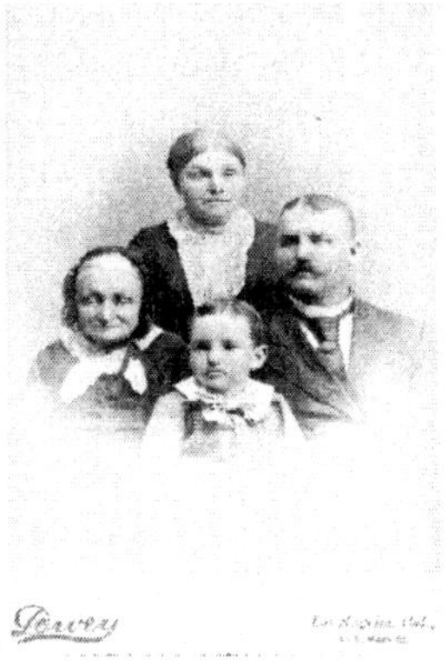

Pictures Left to Right -Top Row (1) Charlotte Hough Maxwell, wife of Archibald (2). John H. Maxwell, eldest son (3) George Bancroft Maxwell, youngest son, my great-great grandfather
Left to Right Bottom Row (1) Marie Maxwell, daughter; (2) Mareta Ruth Maxwell with her husband, Frank; and (3) Charlotte Maxwell; her mother, Magdalena Cook; Samuel Maxwell (middle son of Archibald); and Joe Maxwell (Samuel's son) taken in California after the move in 1881.

EPILOGUE:
Life after Service

After his service ended, Archibald resumed his medical practice in Davenport on the corner of Second Street and Main Street.[474] His transition back to a civilian medical practice went smoothly. He was "welcomed by his old friends who had not forgotten him, together with many new ones added; and his services became in constant demand by rich and poor, and the one was served as well as the other."[475] Through his medical practice, he earned a good living, making a reported income in 1865 of $1,543 for income tax purposes, as published in the local *Davenport Daily Gazette*.[476]

While Archibald transitioned to civilian life again in 1864, the war still raged on touching the lives of many families. Archibald's family was no different. Archibald's brother-in-law, John Cook Jr., fell gravely ill, while serving as an Assistant Surgeon for a Union army expedition into Arkansas in July 1864. He returned to Archibald's Davenport home in the hope that Archibald and his family might once again bring him back from the brink. It was not meant to be, and he died on December 13, 1864, probably of tuberculosis, or a reoccurrence of the lung infection that had nearly killed him in the fall of 1862. It must have been a tough blow. John Cook Jr. was young and a recent graduate of the medical college in Keokuk where Archibald himself had taught him.

Despite the tragic loss of one family member, Archibald and his family had a new bundle of joy born to them in 1864. Ten months after he returned from his trip, He and his wife had a son; George Bancroft Maxwell. Their other children—John H., Marie, Mareta, and Samuel—all grew to adulthood in Davenport.

After the end of Civil War, Archibald had the opportunity to seek elected public office. He remained popular within the state for his service in the war. In 1867, there was a whisper campaign to have him run for governor of Iowa in 1868.[477] Archibald put a stop to it. While the statement comes from the editor of the paper, Archibald likely made clear that he was not interested. He remained focused on his family and medicine.

Although he was not interested in a public leadership role, Archibald continued to be a leader in the Davenport medical community. He served on the Board of Health for the City of Davenport in 1866.[478] He was a consulting surgeon and director of Mercy Hospital. He also assisted Annie Wittenmyer with the founding of her Soldiers' Orphans' home in Davenport and was its doctor.[479] He was a charter member of the Iowa-Illinois District Central Association, a medical society. He served in various executive positions in the Scott County, and Iowa State Medical Societies and Iowa-Illinois District Central Association.[480] Over the years, he also helped young physicians get started, taking many of them as apprentices in his office.

When a cholera epidemic broke out in 1873, he stepped up to lead the medical community of Davenport.[481] That year, cholera swept up and down the Mississippi River Valley stalking its victims. In Davenport, the cholera burned through an impoverished part of Davenport populated with immigrant Danes. For ten days harrowing days, the medical community fought to contain the spread. Archibald took 30 cases.[482] He took more cases than any other doctor in town reported taking. Despite the larger volume of patients, he had a lower reported mortality rate than any other doctor in town.[483] He also led efforts to compile Davenport's report to the U.S. Congress on the Cholera Epidemic of 1873, which Mr. Farquharson revised for final submission.[484]

By the 1880s, Archibald's health was in decline. As he did back in 1852 when he moved to Iowa, Archibald travelled a bit in the Southwest before his move to California. In 1882, he took a trip to the Southwest and decided to move to California. He found the dryer air in the Southwest helped his lung ailment. Archibald invested in a mine, whether this adventure was any more successful than his other business ventures is not known. In 1883, he bought a fruit farm in Los Angeles County and moved there with his three living sons—John, Samuel, and George. By then, his daughters Marie and Mareta had married doctors. Marie remained in Davenport with her husband, Dr. A. W. Bowman. Mareta moved to Pennsylvania with her husband, Dr. Ramsey.

In March 1884, Archibald went out on a house call 40 miles away to treat patients that had fallen ill. When he returned home, he fell ill and never recovered. On March 13, 1884, he died in the company of his family in California. His body was returned to Davenport, where it was laid to rest. The city and the members of his profession honored him with extensive obituaries and memoriam, which testified to the lasting good will and feeling that the people of Davenport had for him as a doctor and a man.

Archibald left a lasting legacy for his descendants and future generations of the Maxwell family and the Davenport community. Archibald brought this branch of the Maxwell family to Davenport in Scott County, Iowa. Many of his descendants still live there today. Also, some of Archibald's descendants followed in his footsteps into a career in medicine; his youngest son, George Bancroft Maxwell, became a very successful doctor in Scott County, Iowa.[485] The Davenport institutions that Archibald helped to establish have continued to play an important role in the community, particularly Mercy Hospital, which is now Genesis Medical Center.

Because Archibald had an impressive list of accomplishments during the Civil War, it is easy to forget that his life before the war involved a merit driven rise from humble circumstances to educated medical doctor and surgeon. He was the tenth child of eleven, who lost his father at age four. His family had no money for his education. With relentless determination and entrepreneurial acumen, he overcame these handicaps to obtain a first rate education. He found a profession in medicine, which he used to benefit society and his family. His life story remains an example to us of what is possible, if one dares to try.

TIMELINE OF EVENTS IN DR. ARCHIBALD S. MAXWELL'S LIFE

June 23, 1818	Born in Tuscarawas County, Ohio
1822	Father, John Maxwell, died
1834	Apprenticed to the printing trade
1836	Moved to Findlay, Ohio as printer for *Findlay Courier*
1837	*Findlay Courier* closed. Archibald joined *Hancock Republican*
1839	Moved to Mansfield, Ohio. Founded Meredith & Maxwell to publish the *Shield and Banner*. Mother, Ruth, died.
1841	Sold, along with his partner, the *Shield and Banner.* Attended Ashland Academy.
1842	Graduated Ashland Academy and pursued career in the law. Became sick, abandoned the law to pursue a career in medicine as a doctor.
1848	Graduated from Western University. Married Charlotte Hough, stepdaughter of his teacher and partner, Dr. John Cook.
1855	Moved with his family from Ohio to Davenport, Iowa.
February 19, 1862	Selected by the citizens of Davenport as part of a group to provide relief to wounded Iowa Soldiers in the aftermath of the Battle at Fort Donelson.
February 20, 1862	Left Davenport with a group for Cairo, Illinois, to assist wounded in the Battle of Fort Donelson.
March 11, 1862	Returned from relief mission, where he had provided medical services in Cairo, Mound City Hospital, Paducah,

	Kentucky, Cincinnati, and on steamboats ferrying wounded between these points.
April 11, 1862	Left on second relief mission to treat Iowa wounded after the Battle of Shiloh.
May 1, 1862	Appointed surgeon in charge of the 8th Ward at the hospital in Hamburg.
May 19, 1862	Appointed regimental surgeon for the 10th Iowa Infantry during the advance on Corinth.
June 19, 1862	Returned to Davenport in ill health.
July 3, 1862	Chaired meeting in Davenport to unite the efforts of Mrs. Annie Wittenmyer's group with the efforts of the Iowa Army State Sanitary Commission led by Reverend Kynett.
July, 1862	Left on third sanitary relief mission to join Colonel Ira Gifford. Passed the Board examination for military surgeons in Keokuk, Iowa.
August, 1862	Appointed surgeon for 13th Iowa Infantry Regiment stationed at Bolivar, Tennessee.
September 18–19, 1862	Appointed First Assistant to John G. T. Holston, medical director for the District of Western Tennessee and Corinth at the Battle of Iuka, Mississippi
October 18, 1862	Appointed Assistant Surgeon U.S.V. stationed at Army Military Hospital in Keokuk, Iowa. Appointed Chair of Physiology and Pathology at the College of Physicians and Surgeons in Keokuk, Iowa.
June 2, 1863	Left Davenport to gather sanitary supplies as he headed downriver to join Iowa State Sanitary Agent Mrs. Annie Wittenmyer at Vicksburg
June 23, 1863	Crossed from Synder's Bluffs near Vicksburg with Annie Wittenmyer.

July 4, 1863	Witnessed with Annie Wittenmyer the surrender at Vicksburg.
August 4, 1863	Returned to Iowa. Met Governor Kirkwood at Iowa City and formally appointed Iowa state sanitary agent.
August 1863	Toured Northeast Iowa and gave speeches on sanitary affairs.
September 1863	Left for inspection of hospitals in the South.
October 8–19, 1863	Inspected hospitals in Memphis and inspected Iowa infantry regiments in the field outside of Memphis.
October 28–November 6, 1863	Visited Vicksburg to inspect hospitals and Iowa infantry regiments in the area
November 6-December 4, 1863	Inspected Hospitals and troops in New Orleans and other parts of Louisiana.
December 9, 1863	Sent his report from Vicksburg after the first leg of his return journey from New Orleans was completed.
February 1864	Questioned in report and investigation in Iowa legislative session.
March 13, 1884	Died in California.

MAPS

Map of Key points of interest in Archibald and the Davenport Relief Committee's Trip after the Battle of Fort Donelson, February 1862.

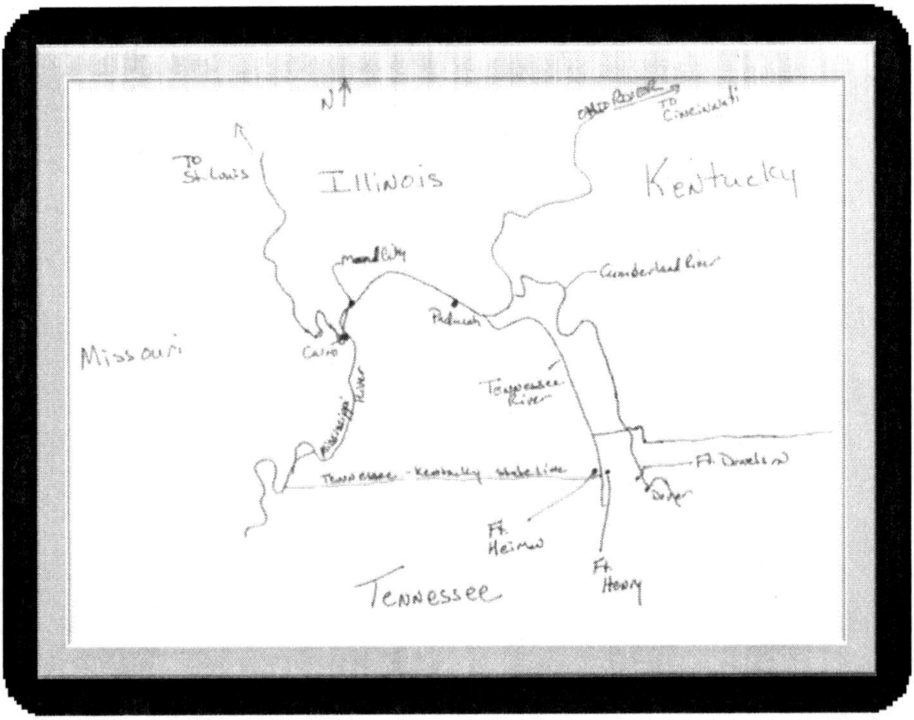

Map of Key Points in the Battle of Shiloh Church, the May 1862 Campaign for Corinth, and the Battle of Iuka.

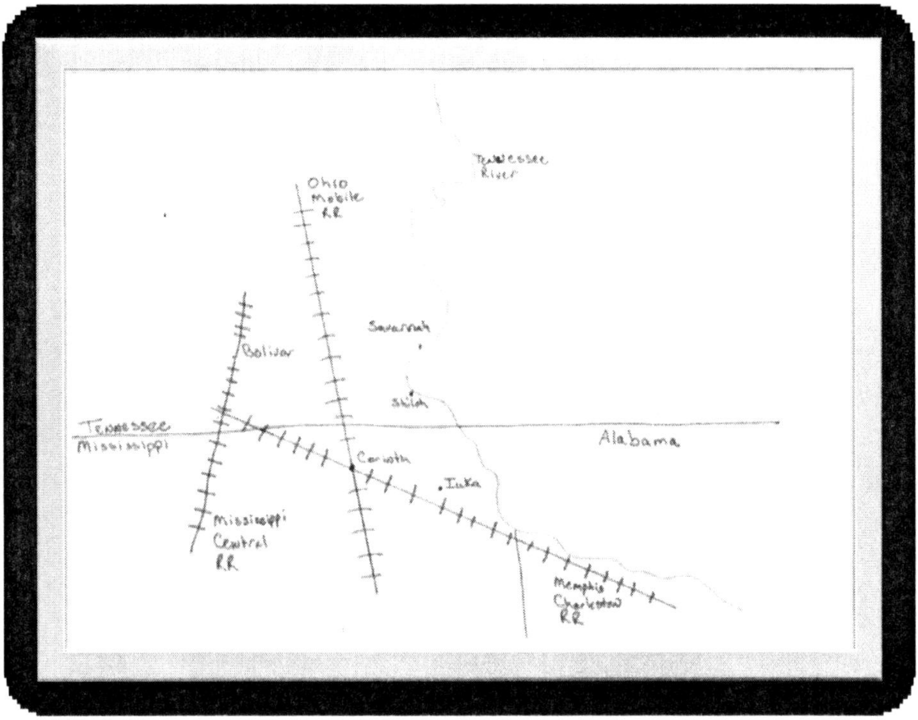

Map of Key Locations in Archibald's Travels and Service during the Civil War

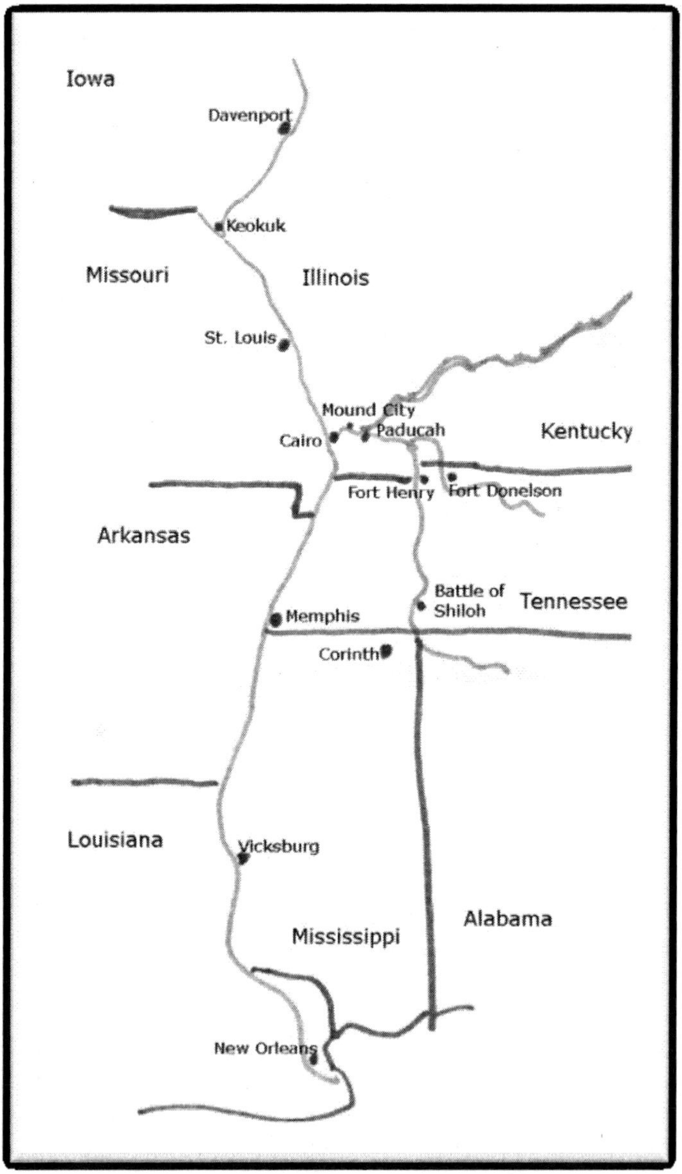

APPENDIX

Statistics gathered by Archibald's November 6, 1863, report to Governor Kirkwood sent from Vicksburg, Mississippi, and in his subsequent December 8, 1863, report addressing troops in Louisiana.

Reg't	Where Camped	Absent Sick	Infantry Present	Men Detached	Officers Sick/Absent/ Present			Signature Strength
4th Cav.	10 miles East of Vicksburg	69	498	88	6	2	7	797
8th Inf.	9 miles East of Vicksburg	87	390	63	2	2	19	524
11th Inf.	2 miles South Vicksburg	10	446	58	1	2	19	613
12th Inf.	9 miles East of Vicksburg	43	246	68	2	2	26	448
13th Inf.	2 miles South of Vicksburg	14	369		3		35	551
15th Inf.	2 miles South of Vicksburg	23	Report not full					
16th Inf.	2 miles South of Vicksburg		Report not full					
35th Inf.	9 miles East of Vicksburg	171	341	75	1	7	16	685
2nd Bat.	At Big Black River Bridge	15	75			1		120

Dr. Maxwell's Abstract of Statistics Obtained from Regimental Record November 1863, as reported in his December 4, 1863, Report.

Date of Visit	Reg't	Where Encamped and Condition	Signature Strength	Men On Duty	Officers' on Duty	Men Sick	Officers ' Sick
Nov. 9th	3rd Inf.	Near Natchez—healthful—very cheerful	512	285	16	16	2

Date of Visit	Reg't	Where Encamped and Condition	Signature Strength	Men On Duty	Officers' on Duty	Men Sick	Officers' Sick
Nov 22nd	21st Inf.	Algiers, La. Headed to Texas—very cheerful	656	456	16	10	1
Nov. 22nd	22nd Inf.	Algiers, La. Headed for Texas (Right wing left for Texas on Nov. 20th in good condition. Left wing left on 22nd in very condition.	627	416	17	9	2
Nov. 26th	24th Inf.	New Iberia, La.—too flat drainage not good—heavy clay subsoil and water from Bayou. Camp equipment bad—blankets and cloths scanty—food good except vegetables are scarce. Men were cheerful. Hospital in good condition. One sick in hospital	599	356	18	7	1
Nov. 26	28th	New Iberia. Same as the 24th as in all their wants. The spirit and general condition of the men and officers are about the same. There is a want of executive ability in the medical department	638	411	33	9	

HOSPITAL DISEASE STATISTICS

Archibald gathered these statistics from hospital records on the number treated for a disease, the treatment used, the number who returned to duty, the number dead, and the number still in hospital in the fall of 1863 from hospitals along the Mississippi River. He passed them along in a November 6th report and a December 9th report to Governor Kirkwood.[486] With regard to the treatments, the handwriting is not the best, and reasonable guesses were made. Where I have no reasonable guess and cannot read the word or abbreviation, I have omitted the word with an ellipsis (...). Archibald wrote Sulph or Sulp., probably short for sulphate. I assume by lead that he referred to acetate lead, which was a drug in the field hospital list during the Civil War.[487] Some of Archibald's numbers do not add up. For example, at Overton, it looks like it should be 146 and not 116. I left his numbers as Archibald wrote them.

# Treated	Disease	Treatment	Returned to Duty	Died	In Hospital
Overton Hospital, Memphis Tennessee—Sept. and Oct. up to the 17th 1863					
116	Acute Diarrhea	Acetate Lead and Opium and Sulphate Zinc	6	2	138
199	Chronic Diarrhea	Acetate Lead and Opiate Linobuithenate	12	9	178
Webster Hospital, Memphis, Tennessee—Sept. and Oct. up to the 17th 1863					
1	Acute Diarrhea	Opium and Quinine			1
160	Chronic Diarrhea	Opium, Bismuth and Zinc	43	13	104
Union Hospital, Memphis, Tennessee—Sept. and Oct. up to the 17th 1863					
7	Acute Diarrhea	No Settled Treatment			7
176	Chronic Diarrhea	Acetate Lead, Opium, Camphor and...	10	49	177
Adams Hospital Memphis Tennessee—Sept. & Oct. up to the 17th 1863					

# Treated	Disease	Treatment	Returned to Duty	Died	In Hospital
39	Acute Diarrhea	Sulphate Zinc and Opium	15	0	24
274	Chronic Diarrhea	Sulphate Zinc and Opium, Quinine and pre diet	37	32	205
Jefferson Hospital Memphis Tennessee—Sept. and Oct. up to the 17th 1863					
40	Acute Diarrhea	Salines—Astringents and Opium	0	2	38
11	Chronic Diarrhea	... Quinine	0	5	6
Washington Hospital, Memphis, Tennessee—Sept.–Oct. 1863					
23	Acute Diarrhea	... and Soda	5	0	18
122	Chronic Diarrhea	Camphor, Acetate Lead, & Opium	21	32	69
Gayoso Hospital, Memphis, Tennessee—Sept.–Oct. 1863					
39	Acute Diarrhea	Nux Vomica (seeds containing Strychnine)	2	8	29
45	Chronic Diarrhea	Nitrate of Silver Zinc ...	3	15	27
Jackson Hospital, Memphis, Tennessee—Sept.–Oct. 1863					
8	Acute Diarrhea	Salines, Opium, Acetate Lead, Camphor	2	1	5
95	Chronic Diarrhea	...	4	34	57
Officer's Hospital, Memphis, Tennessee—Sept.–Oct. 1863					
0	Acute Diarrhea	Salines, ...			
39	Chronic Diarrhea	Salines, Sulphate Zinc and Quinine	11	7	21
Church Hospital, Memphis, Tennessee—Sept.–Oct. 1863					
20	Chronic Diarrhea	Salines, Strychnine , Constitutional Diet	15	3	2

# Treated	Disease	Treatment	Returned to Duty	Died	In Hospital
7	Encephalitis	Local Application Lab sol. Chloride soda ... [3] Tonics and per diet	4	2	1
23	Gangrene	Local solution pre Bromine and Chloride Solution Const. Yeast, Tonics, stringent and pre diet	5	9	9
McPherson Hospital, Vicksburg, Mississippi—Sept.–Oct. 1863 (Visited Oct. 30, 1863)					
36	Acute Diarrhea	Salines, ... and Soda Quinine	2		34
14	Chronic Diarrhea	Salines, ..., Strychnine	1	4	9
32	Dysentery	Salines, ..., Strychnine	3	5	24
Confederate Hospital No. 1, Vicksburg, Mississippi—Oct. 1863 (Visited Oct. 30, 1863)					
27	Acute Diarrhea	Salines, ... Quinine and Opium	2	1	24
50[1]	Chronic Diarrhea	Salines ... Strychnine, Sulphate	8	4	49
7[1]	Dysentery	Oil ..., Acetate Lead and Opium	1	3	6
Confederate Hospital No. 2, Vicksburg, Mississippi—Oct. 1863 (Visited Oct. 30, 1863)					
58	Acute Diarrhea	Salines, ... Soda, Quinine	20		38
48	Chronic Diarrhea	Salines, Acetate Lead and Opium	7	13	48
38	Dysentery	Oil ... Acetate Lead, Strychnine	9	3	26
Confederate Hospital No. 3, Vicksburg, Mississippi—Oct. 1863 (Visited Oct. 30, 1863)					
60	Acute Diarrhea	Oil ... Bitters	14	2	44
53	Chronic Diarrhea	Oil ... Soda Tonics	30	3	20
22	Dysentery	Oil ...,Tonics	7	4	9

# Treated	Disease	Treatment	Returned to Duty	Died	Sick Inst	In Hospital
11th Infantry in Camp 2 Miles South of Vicksburg Record Treatment for October 1863						
16	Acute Diarrhea	Bd. Mass. Saline, … Quinine	9		3	4
10	Chronic Diarrhea	Salines … and Soda Acid mixture, Strychnine	6		4	
42	Dysentery	Salines … … Ammonia, Quinine and Morphine	30		7	5
13th Infantry in Camp 2 Miles South of Vicksburg Record Treatment for October 1863						
20	Diarrhea	Salines …, Sulphate Zinc, Opium	14	2	4	
17	Dysentery	Salines, Opium, Laxatives, and Tonics, and Fowler's Solution was frequently given after or with Quinine	13	1	3	
15th Infantry in Camp 2 Miles South of Vicksburg Record Treatment for October 1863						
40	Acute Diarrhea	… Salines, Opium, Tonics	30	2	2	8
44	Chronic Diarrhea	… … …, Opium, Acetate Lead-Zinc	28	2	12	6
61	Dysentery	…;…	40	2	13	6
16th Infantry in Camp 2 Miles South of Vicksburg Record Treatment for October 1863						
42	Acute Diarrhea	Treatment Not Reported	20		17	5
47	Chronic Diarrhea	Treatment Not Reported	21	1	21	4
62	Dysentery	Treatment Not Reported	36	2	18	6
2nd Iowa Battery Visited Camp on Big Black River Bridge November 4, 1863,						

# Treated	Disease	Treatment	Returned to Duty	Died	Sick Inst	In Hospital
Treatment for September and October 1863						
29	Diarrhea	..., Salines, Opium, Tonics	27			2
28	Dysentery	..., Salines, Opium, Sulphate, ...	26			2

# Treated	Disease	Treatment	Gen. Hospital	Returned to Duty	Died	Sick Inst	Regiment Hospital
8th Infantry in Camps 9 Miles East of Vicksburg on Clear Creek 9 Miles East of Vicksburg Visited on November 5, 1863, Treatment for Sept. and Oct. 1863							
8	Acute Diarrhea	Salines, ...Opium, Tonics, Bismuth		7		1	
1	Chronic Diarrhea	Salines, ... Opium, Astringents prohibited					1
57	Dysentery	Salines, ..., Quinine, ...	3	50	2	1	1
263	Fever	...., Bitters	9	244	2	5	3
12th Infantry in Camps 9 Miles East of Vicksburg on Clear Creek 9 Miles East of Vicksburg Visited on November 5, 1863, Treatment for Sept. and Oct. 1863							
34	Acute Diarrhea	Salines, Opium and Astringents	3	26	1	1	3
3	Chronic Diarrhea	Salines, Opium and Astringents, Tonics and Acids					
2	Dysentery	Salines, Opium and Astringents, Tonics and Acids		2			
149	Fever	...- Tonics and Laxatives	9	132	3	4	1
35th Infantry in Camps 9 Miles East of Vicksburg on Clear Creek 9 Miles East of Vicksburg Visited on November 5, 1863, Treatment for Sept. and Oct. 1863							
44	Acute Diarrhea	Opium, Astringents, Acids	5	21	1	4	3
6	Chronic Diarrhea	... Opium, Acetate Lead		3	3		
57	Dysentery	...	4	44	7		2

# Treated	Disease	Treatment	Gen. Hospital	Returned to Duty	Died	Sick Inst	Regiment Hospital
213	Fever	Treatment Not Reported	115	92	4		2
4th Cavalry in Camps 9 Miles East of Vicksburg on Clear Creek 9 Miles East of Vicksburg Visited on November 5, 1863, Treatment for Sept. and Oct. 1863							
61	Diarrhea	Salines, ..., Opium, Quinine and Acids	5	45		1	
50	Dysentery	... Soda ... ..., Opium, Quinine and Acids	5	44			1
258	Fever	..., Fowler's Solution	110	243	3		2

Hospital Camps in the City of New Orleans, Louisiana Statistics Gathered By Archibald in November 1863

Date	Disease	No. Treated	Treatment and Diet	Discharged	Returned to Duty	Died	In Hospital
U.S. Barracks Hospital							
July	Acute Diarrhea	21	Salines and Opium ...	1	8	1	10
July	Chronic Diarrhea	165	No settled plan—change of air better than medication	6	30	27	76
July	Dysentery	18	Same as Acute Diarrhea		6	4	6
Aug	Acute Diarrhea	13	Salines and Opium ...		6		6
Aug	Chronic Diarrhea	135	No settled plan—change of air better than medication	6	35		25
Aug	Dysentery	11	Same as Acute Diarrhea		4	1	5
Sept.	Acute Diarrhea	7	Salines and Opium ...		4		3
Sept.	Chronic Diarrhea	77	No settled plan—change of air better than medication			59	8
Sept.	Dysentery	3	Same as Acute Diarrhea			3	
Oct.	Acute	6	Salines and Opium ...		3		3

Date	Disease	No. Treated	Treatment and Diet	Discharged	Returned to Duty	Died	In Hospital
	Diarrhea						
Oct.	Chronic Diarrhea	51	No settled plan—change of air better than medication	4	6	30	8
Oct.	Dysentery	6	Same as Acute Diarrhea		1	1	2
May & June	Wounded	196	Water dressing supporting treatment and diet	10	26	8	52
May & June	Wounded	6	Amputations	6			
From Jan.	All cases	3135				421	396
			Convalescent Camps of 13th Army Corps 1st Battalion				
Nov	All Diseases	200	Medication simple diet fair exercise moderate camp duty	10	40		150
			Convalescent Camps of 13th Army Corps 2nd Battalion				
Nov	All Diseases	350	Medication rational, diet select and liberal. Camp duty. Horseback exercises for Chronic Diarrhea cases. Selected amusements.	10	65		275
			University Hospital				
Sept	Acute Diarrhea	13	... sedatives, rest, ... vegetables and diet		10		3
Sept	Chronic Diarrhea	61	...Tonics, Sedatives, modest exercise	5	9	24	18
Sept	Acute Dysentery	19	Salines, Tonics, rest, bland diet and drink	2	8	4	5
Sept	Chronic Dysentery	2	...Turpentine, bland diet, Tonics			2	
Sept	Anemia	31	Free air and light, Mineral Tonics, nutritious food—moderate exercise	2	10		19

Date	Disease	No. Treated	Treatment and Diet	Discharged	Returned to Duty	Died	In Hospital
Sept	Rheumat -ism	16	Salines, Tonics, Fullers Treatment, ... Salts locally applied	1	6		9
Sept	Wounds	150	Free air, plain dressing, nutritious diet	Results not reported			
			St. James Hospital				
July	Acute Diarrhea	14	Salines, Opium, Camphor Ipecac	1	7	2	4
July	Chronic Diarrhea	45	Oak Orchard Mineral water in cases where ... has but first evidenced itself.... Creosote is highly recommended by Dr. Smith in alternative cases also he properly advises free air and diet	5	6	10	22
Aug	Acute Diarrhea	51	Same	1	24	1	20
Aug	Chronic Diarrhea	46	Same	6	40	13	25
Sept.	Acute Diarrhea	75	Same	2	45		20
Sept.	Chronic Diarrhea	31	Same	4	8	11	6
Oct.	Acute Diarrhea	47	Same		20	1	20
Oct.	Chronic Diarrhea	40	Same		8	15	16
3 mths	Wounds	141		14	83	14	41
3 mths	Wounds	13	Amputations	4		4	5
3 mths	All Cases	495				23	136
			Corps Hospital of the 13th Army Corps				
Sept	Chronic	200	Opium Acetate Lead,	4	26	46	100

Date	Disease	No. Treated	Treatment and Diet	Discharged	Returned to Duty	Died	In Hospital
	Diarrhea		Camphor ...				
Oct	All Classes	2112	Distinct assignments defective as are the hygiene—ventilation not good—classification not regarded			200	300
Nov	All Classes	1099			856	65	560
Hospital in and Encampments Near New Iberia, Louisiana 24th Iowa Infantry							
Sept.	Acute Diarrhea	19	... Chlorate Potash ...		19		
Sept.	Chronic Diarrhea	3	Opium and Quinine ... Soda Tonics—liberal diet and moderate exercise horseback		2		1
Sept.	Dysentery	10	Salines and Calomel Turpentine ... Good diet		8		2
Oct.	Diarrhea	2			2		
Oct.	Dysentery	3			2		1
28th Infantry							
Sept.	Acute Diarrhea	15	Acute Diarrhea—Salines, Opium, Quinine and Camphor Chronic Diarrhea ... Zinc, Opium, ... Turpentine and Whiskey Diet moderate bland drinks rest Acute Dysentery—Salines, Calomel, Opium Chronic—same as Chronic Diarrhea. Diet moderate bland drinks rest		15		
Sept.	Chronic Diarrhea	6			6		
Sept.	Dysentery	17			10		6
Oct.	Acute Diarrhea	11			9		2
Oct.	Chronic Diarrhea	3			1	1	1
Oct.	Dysentery	2			2		
U.S. General Hospital at New Iberia, Louisiana							
Nov	Diarrhea	58	... Soda, Opium, Acetate of Lead		18	10	20
From	All Cases	631	But few bad cases treated	18	384	23	136

Date	Disease	No. Treated	Treatment and Diet	Discharged	Returned to Duty	Died	In Hospital
Oct			250 sent to New Orleans				
U.S. General Hospital at Franklin, Louisiana							
From Oct	All Diseases	350	Treatment and Hygiene arrangements and general comforts good …. 110 sent to New Orleans		75	20	100
U.S. Marine Hospital—New Orleans							
July	Acute Diarrhea	10			7		3
July	Chronic Diarrhea		Surgeon expresses his want of confidence in any medication for Chronic Diarrhea but use Opium, Tonics, …. And Astringents a restricted diet … but little … diet allowed. Acute Diarrhea, Dysentery … Salines and Quinine. Chronic Dysentery …. And Turpentine Local Application Iodine to abdomen but very little attention to … exercise or amusements	2	30	44	8
July	Dysentery	3			3		
Aug	Acute Diarrhea	15			10		5
Aug	Chronic Diarrhea	78		2	26	29	12
Aug	Dysentery	13			8	2	3
Sept.	Acute Diarrhea	39			8	2	15
Sept.	Chronic Diarrhea	128		6	46	35	30
Sept.	Dysentery	14			5	3	7
Oct.	Acute Diarrhea	10			5	1	4
Oct.	Chronic Diarrhea	56		2	10	38	6
Oct.	Dysentery	4				3	1
Oct.	Typhoid Fever	25	Reject Tonics and … rest and diet		2	21	2
Oct.	Diphtheria	10	Zinc, … Tonic, Strychnine		3	5	2
3 mths	Gangrene	20	… Tonics and Astringents local Nitric Acid and not used Bromine	Results not reported			
	All cases					493	444

Date	Disease	No. Treated	Treatment and Diet	Discharged	Returned to Duty	Died	In Hospital
			St. Louis Hospital				
Sept.	Diarrhea	57	For Chronic Diarrhea—Opium, Bismuth Tonic stimulants, change of air free diet—discard Astringent	4	12	12	25
Sept.	Dysentery	4				3	1
Oct.	Diarrhea	19		2	12		5
Oct.	Typhoid Fever	12	Ammonia, Tonics rest and nutritious diet		3	3	6
	Wounds	105	Discards excretions. Conservative treatment in the furthest extent preserved.	16	30	9	50
	All Cases	1296	The medication and ... arrangements rather imperfect. The general hygiene condition very good. The female nurses are mostly from citizens of foreign birth			164	319

BIBLIOGRAPHY

MANUSCRIPT COLLECTIONS AND PRIVATE PAPERS

The Annie Wittenmyer Papers, State Historical Society of Iowa.

The Hospital Correspondence, State Historical Society of Iowa.

The Adjutant General's General Correspondence, State Historical Society of Iowa.

The Maxwell Family Papers (copies on file with the author)

Maxwell Family Book, Chapter V by Maxwell, Gary, (unpublished manuscript).

Orphan Court Records, Adams County, Pennsylvania for Estate of James Maxwell 1799–1801

BOOKS AND ARTICLES CONSULTED

Adams, George Worthington. *Doctors in Blue: The Medical History of the Union Army in the Civil War*. New York: Henry Schumen, Inc. 1952. Reprint, Baton Rouge: Louisiana State University Press, 1996.

Arnold, James R. *Grant Wins the War Decision at Vicksburg*. New York: John Wiley & Sons, Inc., 1997.

Atkinson, Williman M.D., ed., *The Physicians and Surgeons of the United States*. Philadelphia: Charles Robson, 1878.

Bolett, Alfred. *Civil War Medicine: Challenge and Triumphs.* :Galen Press, 2002.

Bowman, John S., executive ed. *The Civil War Almanac*. New York: W.H. Smith Publishers, Inc., 1983.

Brinton, John H. *Personal Memoirs of John H. Brinton, Major and Surgeon U.S.V. 1861–1865*. New York: The Neal Publishing Company, 1914.

Cantwell, A. W., M.D. "In Memoriam of A.S. Maxwell M.D. To the President and Members of the Scott County Medical Society." *The Iowa State Medical Reporter* Vol. 1 No. 1 pgs.137-139, July 1883.

Chesson, Michael B., Editor, *The Journal of a Civil War Surgeon/J. Franklin Dryer*: University of Nebraska Press, 2003.

Child, William, Editor, *Letters from a Civil War Surgeon: The Letters of Dr. William Child of the 5th New Hampshire Volunteers*: Polar Bear and Co., 2001.

D., Amy "Not Gone Before His Time: The Adventures of Civil War Captain Harry B. Doolittle." Primary Selections from Special Collections, Richardson-Sloane Special Collections Blog for Davenport Public Library, Posted March 9, 2012, available at http://blogs.davenportlibrary.com/sc/2012/03/09/not-gone-before-his-time-the-adventures-of-civil-war-captain-harry-b-doolittle/.Downer, Harry E. *History of Davenport and Scott County, Iowa Illustrated*, Vol. 1, part 2. Chicago: The S. J. Clarke Publishing Company, 1910.

Evans, David Morier. *The History of the Commercial Crisis 1857–58 and the Stock Exchange Panic of 1859*. London: Groombridge and Sons, 1859.

Fatout, Paul, Editor, *Letters of Civil War Surgeon*: Purdue Research Foundation, 1996.

Forman, J.G.. *The Western Sanitary Commission; a Sketch of its Origins, History, Labors for the Sick and Wounded of the Western Armies and Aid Given to Freedmen and Union Refugees with Incidents of Hospital Life.* St. Louis: R.P. Studley & Co., 1864.

Fullbrook, Earl S.. "Relief Work in Iowa During the Civil War." *Iowa Journal of History and Politics*, Vol. XVI No. 2, Benjamin Shambaugh, ed., Iowa City: The State Historical Society, April 1918.

Goodrich, Frank B. *The Munificence, Self-Sacrifice and Patriotism of the American People During the War For the Union*. New York: Derby and Miller, 1865.

Grant, Ulysses S. *Personal Memoirs of U.S. Grant*. Two Volumes in One. Connecticut: Konecky & Konecky, 1999.

Greiner, James M., Coryell, Janet L., and Smither, James, Editors, *A Surgeon's Civil War The Letters and Diary of Daniel M. Holt, M.D.* : The Kent State University Press, 1994.

Iowa Sanitary Commission. "Report of the Iowa Sanitary Commission from Its Organization October 13, 1861 to the Close of Its Service By the Transfer of Its Work to the New Commission December 1, 1863 To His Excellency

Samuel J. Kirkwood, Governor of Iowa." Davenport Publishing House of Luse, Lane & Co., 1864.

Kynett, Reverend A. J and Magoun, Reverend George of the Army Sanitary Commission of the State of Iowa. "Report on the Condition of the Iowa Camps and Hospitals." Lyons, Iowa: Beers & Eaton, Mirror Office, January 1862.

Lathrop, H. W. *The Life and Times of Samuel J. Kirkwood, Iowa's War Governor*. Chicago: Regan Printing House, 1893.

Leonard, Elizabeth D. "'Men Did Not Take To The Musket More Commonly Than Women To the Needle': Annie Wittenmyer and Soldiers' Aid." *Yankee Women: Gender Battles in the Civil War*. New York: W.W. Norton & Company, 1994. Reprint by permission, Bergman, Marvin, ed. *Iowa History Reader*, Iowa City: University of Iowa Press, 1996.

Lyftogt, Kenneth, *Left for Dixie: The Civil War Diary of John Rath*. Iowa City: Camp Pope Bookshop, 2004.

Maxwell, A. Dr. and Wittenmyer, Annie, State Sanitary Agents, *Sanitary Circular,* July 30, 1863.

Maxwell, Dr. Archibald S. "Dr. Maxwell's Report." Report of the Adjutant General and Acting Quartermaster General of the State of Iowa January 1, 1863 to January 11, 1864." Des Moines: F.W. Palmer, State Printer, 1864.

Meacham, Jon. *American Lion: Andrew Jackson in the White House.* New York: Random House, 2008.

McDevitt, Theresa R. "'A Melody Before Unknown': the Civil War Experiences of Mary and Amanda Shelton," *The Annals of Iowa*, V. 63 Number 2, pg. 109 (State Historical Society of Iowa Spring 2004), 109.

Newberry, J. S., Dr. *The U.S. Sanitary Commission in the Valley of the Mississippi, During the War of the Rebellion, 1861–1866*. Cleveland: Fairbanks, Benedict & Co. 1871.

Stille, Charles J. *History of the United States Sanitary Commission Being the General Report of its Work During the War of the Rebellion*. New York: Hurd and Houghton, 1868.

Twombly, V.P., Captain. *The Second Iowa Infantry At Fort Donelson, February 15, 1862 Together with an Outline History of the Regiment from its Organization at Keokuk, Iowa, May 27, 1861 to Final Discharge at Davenport, Iowa, July 20, 1865*. Des Moines: Plain Talking Printing House, 1901.

United States House of Representatives, 43d Congress, 2nd Session, *The Cholera Epidemic of 1873 in the United States*, Ex. Doc. No. 95, Washington D.C., Government Printing Office, 1875.

Wilbur, C. Keith. *Civil War Medicine*.: The Globe Pequote Press, 1998.

Woodward, J. J. Ass. Surgeon U.S.A. *Medical and Surgical History of the War of the Rebellion, Part 1, Vol. 1 Medical History*. Washington D.C.: Government Printing Office, 1870.

Wittenmyer, Annie. *Under the Guns: A Woman's Reminiscences of The Civil War*. Boston: E.B. Stillings & Co., 1895.

_______Journal of the House of Representative at the Extra Session of the Ninth General Assembly of the State of Iowa, which convened at the Capital in Des Moines, on Wednesday, the Third Day of September A.D. 1862, Des Moines: F.W. Palmer, State Printer,1862.

_______Journal of the House of Representatives of the Tenth Assembly of the State of Iowa, Which Convened at the Capital in Des Moines, January 11, 1864, Des Moines: F.W. Palmer, State Printer, 1864.

_______Journal of the Senate of the Tenth Assembly of the State of Iowa, Which Convened at the Capital in Des Moines, January 11, 1864, Des Moines: F.W. Palmer, State Printer,1864.

_______*United States Biographical Dictionary and Portrait Gallery of Eminent and Self-Made Men, Iowa Volume*. Chicago and New York: Chicago and New York American Biographical Publishing Company, 1878.

_______*History of Scott County, Iowa*. Chicago: Inter-State Publishing Co., 1882.

PERIODICALS CONSULTED

Annals of Iowa
American Medical Times

Burlington Weekly Hawk-Eye
Cedar Falls Gazette
Davenport Daily Gazette
Davenport Democrat and Leader
Davenport Democrat and News
Findlay Courier
Holmes County Farmer
Holmes County Republican
Iowa State Medical Reporter
Maumee Express

ILLUSTRATION CREDITS

Grateful acknowledgement is made to the following for permission to reprint photos and illustrations:

Photos of Archibald S. Maxwell and family members: The Maxwell Family
Photos of the Letter Appointing Archibald S. Maxwell, Assistant Surgeon of Volunteers, October 18, 1862, the Ohio Militia Certificate, the Replica of Shiloh Church, and the railroad crossing in Corinth, Mississippi: Mary Christenson.
Photo of the College of Physicians and Surgeons 1860: The University of Iowa
Map of the Vicksburg Siege Lines, Records of the Adjutant General, Sanitary Agents Reports, Civil War (series), State Historical Society of Iowa, Des Moines.

NOTES

[1] If you find the general topic interesting, you might start with George Washington Adams's *Doctors in Blue*, a classic covering the medical history of the Union Army. You can find additional information on the soldiers' relief in Iowa by consulting the excellent book *Yankee Women* by Elizabeth Leonard. Other books address the medicine provided and advances in medicine, such as *Civil War Medicine* by C. Keith Wilbur (Old Saybrook: The Globe Pequote Press, 1998) and *Civil War Medicine: Challenge and Triumphs* by Alfred Bolett (Tuscon: Galen Press, 2002).

[2] J. G. Forman, *The Western Sanitary Commission; a Sketch of its Origins, History, Labors for the Sick and Wounded of the Western Armies and Aid Given to Freedmen and Union Refugees with Incidents of Hospital Life*, St. Louis: R. P. Studley & Co.,1864, 3–7. (Hereafter Forman, *The Western Sanitary Commission).* The incident discussed in the prologue is discussed extensively.

[3] Ibid.

[4] Ibid.

[5] Ibid.

[6] Ibid.

[7] Ibid.

[8] Dr. J. S. Newberry, *The U.S. Sanitary Commission in the Valley of the Mississippi, During the War of the Rebellion, 1861–1866,*18. *(*Hereafter Newberry, *The U.S. Sanitary Commission in the Valley of the Mississippi)*

[9] George Worthington Adams, *Doctors in Blue: The Medical History of the Union Army in the Civil War.* New York: Henry Schumen, Inc. 1952. Reprint, Baton Rouge: Louisiana State University Press, *1996*, 194. (Hereafter Adams, *Doctors in Blue*).

[10] *United States Biographical Dictionary and Portrait Gallery of Eminent and Self-Made Men*, Iowa Volume, (Chicago and New York: American Biographical Publishing Company, 1878. (Hereafter referred to as *Biographical Dictionary of 1878*), 579–581.

As noted in the preface, the persons listed in the book provided "requisite information" which likely means that the individuals noted provided some or all of the information in the biographical sketches.

[11] The trek took years. Archibald's eldest brother, Samuel, and two older sisters, Mary and Jane, were born in Adams County and York County, Pennsylvania, in 1795, 1799, and 1801, respectively. John's father, James, died in 1799. James died without a will. The estate, including two farms, was sold in 1801 and divided among James' six children. See Orphan Court Records, Adams County, Pennsylvania for Estate of James Maxwell 1799–1801. John's share likely was the source of funds for his move and purchase of land in Ohio.

[12] In 1804, John and Ruth had a son, Robert, who was born in Jefferson County, Ohio. Gary Maxwell, "Chapter V," *Maxwell Family Book*, (self published). John and Ruth also had a daughter, Isabel, in 1809 in Jefferson County. John Maxwell paid taxes on land in that county in 1806 and 1807.

[13] Archibald's older brother John is the first sibling born in Tuscarawas County in 1811, suggesting that the family had moved.

[14] -----,Died, "Obituary of Margaret Rainsburg," *Holmes County Farmer*, March 7, 1861. Col. 3, 3.. The same obituary appears in the *Holmes County Republican*, Obituary Notices, March 21, 1861, Col. 3, 3.

[15] The obituaries of A. S. Maxwell's brothers Bezaleel and Abner Maxwell all mention the move to Berlin in Holmes County in 1824. -------, "Obituary of Abner Maxwell," *Holmes County Farmer*, November 24, 1887, 3; ------ "Obituary of Bezaleel Maxwell," *Holmes County Farmer*, June 17, 1875.

[16] *Biographical Dictionary of 1878*, 579–580.

[17] Ibid; "A List of Letters," *Findlay Courier*, January 10, 1837, Col. 3, 3, which lists Archibald Maxwell as one of Findlay residents who has a letter left at the post office on December 31, 1836.

[18] Jon Meacham, *American Lion Andrew Jackson in the White House* (New York: Random House, 2008), 210; 335.

---

[19] *Biographical Dictionary of 1878*, 579–580; *Maumee Express*, November 25, 1837, Col. 2, 2, which states "We learn from the Miami of the Lake that the *Findlay Courier* has expired. In the *Courier*, Democracy have lost one of the most able, powerful, elaborate and original of their advocates."

[20] *Biographical Dictionary of 1878*, 579–580; *Maumee Express*, February 10, 1838, Col. 3, 2, "We have received the first number of a very neatly executed paper entitled the *Hancock Republican*, published at Findlay, Ohio by A. F. Miriam. The editor appears to be a man of talent, whose object is that of laboring for the welfare of the Whig party, the place, and the country surrounding him. May success attend him."

[21] *Biographical Dictionary of 1878*, 579–580. In the *Biographical Dictionary*, it was described as follows: "In 1837, being a master workman, he was employed as a foreman of the "Whig" office for one year; there he enjoyed the society of a cultivated gentleman and lady (Mr. and Mrs. Marion [sic]), who gave him great assistance in the study of Latin, Greek, and French during his hours of recreation."

[22] John Meredith, "Letter to Patrons of the Shield and Banner," *Shield and Banner*, June 24, 1841, Col. 1, 3.

[23] Ibid.

[24] H. W. Lathrop, *The Life and Times of Samuel J. Kirkwood, Iowa's War Governor* (Chicago: Regan Printing House: 1893), 20.

[25] *Biographical Dictionary of 1878*, 579–580.

[26] Ibid.

[27] A. S. Maxwell's mentor, Mr. Brinkerhoff, was a Free-Soil democrat and supposedly was one of the Democrats responsible for the Wilmot Proviso that limited expansion of slavery into the lands seized in the war from Mexico. A. S. would later turn down the opportunity to take a nomination for public office because the Democratic platform on slavery was not compatible with his beliefs. *Biographical Dictionary of 1878*, 579–580.

[28]John Meredith, "Letter to Patrons of the Shield and Banner," *Shield and Banner*, June 24, 1841, Col. 1, 3.

[29] John Meredith and A. S. Maxwell, *Shield and Banner*, March 18, 1841, Col. 2, 3, reporting the results of the Mechanics Meeting on Saturday, March 6, 1841, noting that A. S. Maxwell was president.

[30] Commission Certificate for A. S. Maxwell's Appointment as Adjutant in the Ohio Militia, dated June 9, 1842, copy with Author.

[31] *Biographical Dictionary of 1878*, 580.

[32] Ibid., 581.

[33] Ibid., 580.

[34] Ibid.

[35] Ibid.,580.

[36] Letter from Reverend A. J. Kynett to Gov. Samuel J. Kirkwood of Iowa, June 21, 1862.

[37] A. W. Cantwell,, M.D. "In Memoriam of A. S. Maxwell M.D. To the President and Members of the Scott County Medical Society," *The Iowa State Medical Reporter*, Vol. 1 No. 1, July 1883, 137–139. (Hereafter Cantwell, *A.S. Maxwell*).

[38] Ibid.

[39] Adams, *Doctors in Blue*, 49.

[40] Ibid; The *Biographical Dictionary of 1878* incorrectly refers to it as Hudson College. A. S. Maxwell was listed as a Student of Western Reserve College in the Medical Department and a graduate in 1847 and 1848 in the online list of student roster for Western Reserve College located at http://morganoh.startlogic.com/WesternReserveCollege.html. Western Reserve College was at the time located in Hudson, Ohio, which is probably where the confusion arises.

[41] Cantwell, *A.S. Maxwell*,138.

[42] *Biographical Dictionary of 1878*, 580.

[43] *History of Scott County, Iowa*. (Chicago: Inter-State Publishing Co., 1882), 668–669.

[44] Cantwell, *A.S. Maxwell*, 138; *Biographical Dictionary of 1878*, 580.

[45] *Biographical Dictionary of 1878*, 580.

[46] David Morier Evans, *The History of the Commercial Crisis 1857–58 and the Stock Exchange Panic of 1859* (Groombridge and Sons, London 1859), 34.

[47] *Biographical Dictionary of 1878*, 580.

[48] "Notice of Sheriff Sale," *Davenport Daily Gazette,* July 8, 1862, Col. 7, 1. Notice of planned sheriff sale of certain real estate property in favor of Lorenzo Schrieker against Samuel Saddorris and A. S. Maxwell to satisfy the debt of $874.97. Sale to take place in August 1862.

[49] Cantwell, *A.S. Maxwell*, 138.

[50] "Advertisement for A. S. Maxwell M.D.," *Davenport Daily Gazette*, December 29, 1855, Col. 3, 1; "Advertisement for A. S. Maxwell M.D.," *Davenport Daily Gazette*, February 11, 1856, Col. 3, 1.

[51] *Biographical Dictionary of 1878*, 580.

[52] Harry E. Downer, *History of Davenport and Scott County, Iowa Illustrated*, Vol. 1 part 2, (Chicago: The S. J. Clarke Publishing Company, 1910), 501.

[53] *History of Scott County, Iowa* (Chicago: Inter-State Publishing Co.,1882), 672.

[54] "Surgical Operation," *Davenport Daily Gazette*, March 27, 1860, Col. 3, 1; "Surgical Operation," *Davenport Daily Gazette*, April 13, 1860, Col. 4, 1.

[55] *Davenport Daily Gazette*, October 6, 1860, Col, 7, 4.

[56] A. S. Maxwell Secretary School Board, "Office of School Board, Davenport April 30, 1859," *Davenport Democrat and Leader*, May 11, 1859. Col. 4, 1.

[57] Th. Saunders, Secretary and Dr. A.S. Maxwell, Pres., "School Meeting," *Davenport Democrat and Leader*, September 26, 1859, Col. 4, 1. At the same meeting where the tax levy was voted down, the community voted to educate African-Americans

(although in a separate school.) "Meeting of the School Board," *Davenport Democrat and Leader*, September 26, 1859, Col. 4, 1. "School Excitement," *Davenport Democrat and Leader*, September 26, 1859, Col. 3, 1.

[58] "The School Meeting, The Public School Sustained, A Large Majority for the Tax," *Davenport Daily Gazette*, Oct. 10, 1859, Col. 3, 1; See also, "The School Board Election Today," *Davenport Daily Gazette*, Oct. 8, 1859, Col. 3, 1. In March of 1860, he was re-elected President of the School Board at Citizen's Meeting by a wide margin on March 5th. However, the Newspaper on March 6th published a correction and listed a new date at which time there would be a vote on a new levy to fund the school and also again for the school board. A. S. Maxwell was not elected at that meeting and due to some controversy the Secretary was also replaced although the accusations were found to be false by the paper. "The School Meeting," *Davenport Daily Gazette*, March 5, 1860, Col. 3, 1; "Election of School Officers," *Davenport Daily Gazette*, March 6, 1860, Col. 3, 1; "Neatly Kept Books," *Davenport Daily Gazette*, March 20, 1860, Col. 2, 1; "Meeting of the New School Board," *Davenport Daily Gazette*, March 21, 1860, Col. 3, 1.

[59] "Died," "Obituary of Margaret Rainsburg," *Holmes County Farmer*, March 7, 1861, Col. 3 . The same obituary appears in the "Obituary Notices," *Holmes County Republican*, March 21, 1861. Col. 3, 3. She survived the surgery fine and appeared to be making a recovery when infection set in and killed her.

[60] Ibid.

[61] Gary Maxwell, "Chapter IV," *Maxwell Family Book* (Manuscript) on file with author, citing death, *Davenport Daily Gazette*, April 22, 1861, reporting death of Elta Margaret on April 20th.

[62] "Obituary Notices: J. M. Cook M.D.," *Holmes Country Republican*, May 30, 1861, 3.

[63] "Death of Dr. John F. Cook," *Holmes County Farmer*, February 2 1865, 3.

[64] L. C. Burwell, "Report of the Davenport Relief Committee," *Davenport Daily Gazette*, Saturday March 8, 1862, 2.

[65] Adams, *Doctors in Blue*, 208–211.

[66] Ibid., 211.

---

[67] Ibid., 4–5.

[68] N.N.T. "14th Iowa Infantry, "Benton Barracks Near St. Louis," *Davenport Daily Gazette*, January 7, 1862; C. C. Park Iowa 12th Regiment Surgeon, "Report," *Davenport Daily Gazette*, January 24, 1862.

[69] "Public Lecture," *Davenport Daily Gazette*, January 17, 1862, 1.

[70] "Minutes of Scott County Medical Society Meeting," *Davenport Daily Gazette*, April 2, 1861,2; "Board of Education Minutes of November 18, 1861 Meeting," *Davenport Daily Gazette*, November 23, 1861, 1.

[71] Charles J. Stille, *United States Sanitary Commission Being the General Report of its Work During the War of Rebellion, 1861-1866.* Cleveland: Fairbanks, Benedict & Co. 1871, 56–64.

[72] Newberry, *The United States Sanitary Commission in the Valley of the Mississippi*, 18.

[73] Ibid.

[74] Both the U.S. Sanitary Commission and the Iowa State Army Sanitary Commission recorded that the Keokuk Ladies Aid Society network worked mainly with the Western Sanitary Commission. Newberry, *The United States Sanitary Commission in the Valley of the Mississippi*, 239. Reverend A. J. Kynett and Reverend George Magoun of the Army Sanitary Commission of the State of Iowa, *Report on the Condition of the Iowa Camps and Hospitals*. Lyons: Beers & Eaton, Mirror Office, January 1862, 9.

[75] Ibid.

[76] Letter from Annie Wittenmyer to Dr. Archibald S. Maxwell, dated August 3, 1863, , Annie Turner Wittenmyer Papers 1861-1901, Special Collections, State Historical Society of Iowa, Des Moines.

[77] Reverend A. J. Kynett and Reverend George Magoun of the Army Sanitary Commission of the State of Iowa, *Report on the Condition of the Iowa Camps and Hospitals* (Lyons: Beers & Eaton, Mirror Office, January 1862), 9.

[78] Ibid.

[79] Elizabeth D. Leonard, "'Men Did Not Take to the Musket More Commonly Than Women To the Needle': Annie Wittenmyer and Soldiers' Aid," *Iowa History Reader*, Bergman, Marvin, ed.,.(Iowa City: University of Iowa Press, 1996). (Hereinafter Leonard, *Annie Wittenmyer and Soldiers' Aid*), 110–111.

[80] Elizabeth D. Leonard, ""Men Did Not Take to the Musket More Commonly Than Women to the Needle': Annie Wittenmyer and Soldiers' Aid. *Yankee Women: Gender Battles in the Civil War.* New York: W.W. Norton & Company, 1994, 56. (Hereafter Leonard, *Yankee Women*.)

[81] Newberry, *The United States Sanitary Commission in the Valley of the Mississippi*, 239.

[82] Iowa Sanitary Commission, *Report of the Iowa Sanitary Commission from Its Organization October 13, 1861 to the Close of Its Service By the Transfer of Its Work to the New Commission December 1, 1863 To His Excellency Samuel J. Kirkwood, Governor of Iowa* (Publishing House of Luse, Lane & Co. Davenport,1864), 3

[83] Ibid.

[84] Leonard, *Annie Wittenmyer and Soldiers' Aid*, 112.

[85] Ibid, at 112–114.

[86] Ibid.

[87] See N.N.T. 14th Iowa Infantry, "Benton Barracks Near St. Louis," *Davenport Daily Gazette*, January 7, 1862; C.C. Park Iowa 12th Regiment Surgeon, "Report," *Davenport Daily Gazette*, January 24, 1862.

[88] Reverend A. J. Kynett and Reverend George Magoun of the Army Sanitary Commission of the State of Iowa, *Report on the Condition of the Iowa Camps and Hospitals* (Lyons: Beers & Eaton, Mirror Office, January 1862) 9.

[89] U. S. Grant, *The Personal Memoirs of Ulysses S. Grant* (Old Saybrook: William S. Konecky & Associates, 1999) 168 (hereafter Grant, *Grant Memoirs*).

[90] Grant, *Grant Memoirs*, 168.

---

[91] Captain V. P. Twombly, *The Second Iowa Infantry At Fort Donelson, February 15, 1862 Together with an Outline History of the Regiment from its Organization at Keokuk, Iowa, May 27, 1861 to Final Discharge at Davenport, Iowa, July 20, 1865* (Des Moines: Plain Talking Printing House, 1901), 10.

[92] Ibid., 13. Reprinting the Report of Major General Charles F. Smith Commanding the 2nd Division at Fort Donelson.

[93] Jules, "From the Iowa 2D Regiment," *Davenport Daily Gazette*, March 8, 1862, Col 3, 2.

[94] "Citizen's Meeting at Le Claire House," *Davenport Daily Gazette*, February 20, 1862, Col. 3, 1.

[95] Grant, *Grant Memoirs*, 177.

[96]Ibid.

[97] Adams, *Doctors in Blue,* 80.

[98] Newberry, *The U.S. Sanitary Commission in the Valley of the Mississippi*, 31–32.

[99] Adams, *Doctors in Blue,* 80.

[100] Dr. Archibald Maxwell, "Report of the Relief Committee Dr. Maxwell's Report," *Davenport Daily Gazette*, March 22, 1862,1.

[101] Ibid.

[102] John Brinton, *Personal Memoirs of John H. Brinton, Major and Surgeon U.S.V. 1861-1865.* (New York: The Neal Publishing Company, 1914), 134. (Hereafter Brinton, *Personal Memoirs of John H. Brinton*)

[103] Dr. Archibald Maxwell, "Report of the Relief Committee Dr. Maxwell's Report," *Davenport Daily Gazette*, March 22, 1862, 1.

[104] Ibid.

[105] Dr. Archibald Maxwell, "Report of the Relief Committee Dr. Maxwell's Report," *Davenport Daily Gazette*, March 22, 1862, 1.

[106] L. C. Burwell, "Report of the Davenport Relief Committee," *Davenport Daily Gazette*, Saturday March 8, 1862, 2.

[107] Dr. Archibald Maxwell, "Report of the Relief Committee Dr. Maxwell's Report," *Davenport Daily Gazette*, March 22, 1862, 1.

[108] Adams, *Doctors in Blue*, 80.

[109] Dr. Archibald Maxwell, "Report of the Relief Committee Dr. Maxwell's Report," *Davenport Daily Gazette*, March 22, 1862, 1.

[110] Ibid.

[111] "False Alarm," *Davenport Democrat and News*, March 24, 1862, 1.

[112] Dr. Archibald Maxwell, "Report of the Relief Committee Dr. Maxwell's Report," *Davenport Daily Gazette*, March 22, 1862, 1.

[113]Ibid.

[114] Ibid.

[115] Brinton, *Personal Memoirs of John H. Brinton*, 45.

[116] Dr. Archibald Maxwell, "Report of the Relief Committee Dr. Maxwell's Report," Davenport Daily Gazette, March 22, 1862, 1

[117] Ibid.

[118] Captain V. P. Twombly, *The Second Iowa Infantry At Fort Donelson, February 15, 1862 Together with an Outline History of the Regiment from its Organization at Keokuk, Iowa, May 27, 1861 to Final Discharge at Davenport, Iowa, July 20, 1865* (Des Moines: Plain Talking Printing House, 1901), 10.

[119] "False Alarm," *Davenport Democrat and News*, March 24, 1862, 1.

[120] Dr. Archibald Maxwell, "Report of the Relief Committee Dr. Maxwell's Report," *Davenport Daily Gazette*, March 22, 1862, 1.

[121] Amy D., "Not Gone Before His Time: The Adventures of Civil War Captain Harry B. Doolittle," *Primary Selections from Special Collections*, Richardson-Sloane Special

Collections Blog for Davenport Public Library, Posted March 9, 2012, available at http://blogs.davenportlibrary.com/sc/2012/03/09/not-gone-before-his-time-the-adventures-of-civil-war-captain-harry-b-doolittle/.

122 "False Alarm," Davenport Democrat and News, March 24, 1862, 1.

123 Jules, "From the Iowa 2D Regiment," *Davenport Daily Gazette*, March 8, 1862, Col. 3, 2.

124 Dr. Archibald Maxwell, "Report of the Relief Committee Dr. Maxwell's Report," *Davenport Daily Gazette*, March 22, 1862, 1.

125 L. C. Burwell, "Report of the Davenport Relief Committee," *Davenport Daily Gazette*, Saturday March 8, 1862, 2.

126 Newberry, *The U.S. Sanitary Commission in the Valley of the Mississippi*, 29.

127 L. C. Burwell, "Report of the Davenport Relief Committee," *Davenport Daily Gazette*, Saturday March 8, 1862, 2.

128 Ibid.

129 Dr. Archibald Maxwell, "Report of the Relief Committee Dr. Maxwell's Report," *Davenport Daily Gazette*, March 22, 1862, 1.

130 Ibid.

131 Ibid.

132 Forman, *The Western Sanitary Commission*, 24.

133 Dr. Archibald Maxwell, "Report of the Relief Committee Dr. Maxwell's Report," *Davenport Daily Gazette*, March 22, 1862, 1.

134 Ibid.

135 Ibid.

136 Ibid.

[137] L. C. Burwell, "Report of the Davenport Relief Committee," Davenport Daily Gazette, Saturday March 8, 1862, 2.

[138] Ibid.

[139] "Aid For Iowa Soldiers," *Davenport Daily Gazette*, April 10, 1862, Morning edition, 1; "Constitution of Scott County Soldiers' Aid Association," *Davenport Daily Gazette*, April 8, 1862, 1.

[140] "Aid For Iowa Soldiers," *Davenport Daily Gazette*, April 10, 1862, Morning edition, 1.

[141] At least in January of 1862, the Davenport ladies aid societies were working with the Keokuk Ladies Aid Society. For more information, please see the January 1862 report. Reverend A. J. Kynett and Reverend George Magoun of the Army Sanitary Commission of the State of Iowa, *Report on the Condition of the Iowa Camps and Hospitals* (Lyons: Beers & Eaton, Mirror Office, January 1862), 9.

[142] "Report of Finance Committee," Davenport Daily Gazette, Friday Morning April 4, 1862,1.

[143]"Aid For Iowa Soldiers," Davenport Daily Gazette, April 10, 1862, Morning edition, 1.

[144] Ibid.

[145] "Report of Finance Committee," *Davenport Daily Gazette*, Friday Morning April 4, 1862,1.

[146] *Davenport Daily Gazette*, March 22, 1862, Morning edition, 1.

[147] "Report of Finance Committee," Davenport Daily Gazette, Friday Morning April 4, 1862,1.

[148] Ibid.

[149] Ibid.

[150] *Davenport Daily Gazette*, April 18, 1862, Morning edition, 1.

[151] *Davenport Daily Gazette*, April 18, 1862, Morning edition, 1.

[152] Grant, *Grant Memoirs*, 200.

[153] *Davenport Daily Gazette*, April 11, 1862, Morning edition, 1.

[154] Dr. Gamble, "Letter from the Relief Commission," *Davenport Daily Gazette*, April 22, 1862, Morning edition, 1.

[155]Dr. Archibald Maxwell and Dr. Gamble, "Surgeons' Report," *Davenport Daily Gazette*, May 9, 1862, Morning edition, 3.

[156] L. C. Burwell, "The Report of L. C. Burwell," *Davenport Daily Gazette,* June 5, 1862, Morning edition, 2.

[157] Letter from Dr. A. S. Maxwell to Governor Kirkwood, June 30, 1862, in Hospital Correspondence, Iowa State Historical Archives.

[158] Dr. Archibald Maxwell and Dr. Gamble, "Surgeons' Report," *Davenport Daily Gazette*, May 9, 1862, Morning edition, 3.

[159] Ibid.

[160] Ibid.

[161] Ibid.

[162] Ibid.

[163] Ibid.

[164] Newberry, *The U.S. Sanitary Commission in the Valley of the Mississippi,* 34–35.

[165] Ibid.

[166] Ibid.

[167] Ibid.

[168] Adams, *Doctors in Blue*, 81. It discusses extensively the effect the course of the battle had on the medical care deficiencies.

[169] Ibid, 39.

[170] L. C. Burwell, "The Report of L.C. Burwell," *Davenport Daily Gazette*, June 5, 1862, Morning edition, 2.

[171] Dr. Archibald Maxwell and Dr. Gamble, "Surgeons' Report," *Davenport Daily Gazette*, May 9, 1862, Morning edition, 3.

[172] Ibid.

[173] Forman, *The Western Sanitary Commission*, 43.

[174] Dr. Gamble, "Letter from the Relief Commission," *Davenport Daily Gazette*, April 22, 1862, Morning edition, 1.

[175] L. C. Burwell, "Report of Mr. L.C. Burwell," *Davenport Daily Gazette*, June 5, 1862, Morning edition, 2.

[176] Letter from Dr. Archibald S. Maxwell to Governor Kirkwood, June 30, 1862, Records of the Adjutant General, Sanitary Agents Reports, Civil War (series), State Historical Society of Iowa, Des Moines.

[177] Dr. Archibald Maxwell and Dr. Gamble, "Surgeons' Report," Davenport Daily Gazette, May 9, 1862, Morning edition, 3.

[178] Annie Wittenmyer, *Under the Guns: A Woman's Reminiscences of The Civil War*. Boston: E.B. Stillings & Co., 1895. (Hereafter Wittenmyer, *Under the Guns*).

[179] Dr. Archibald Maxwell and Dr. Gamble, "Surgeons' Report," Davenport Daily Gazette, May 9, 1862, 3.

[180] Ibid.

[181] Afterward, Governor Harvey's wife devoted herself to the cause of the wounded and sick soldiers in the Civil War.

[182] Dr. Archibald Maxwell and Dr. Gamble, "Surgeons' Report," Davenport Daily Gazette, May 9, 1862, 3.

[183] Ibid.

[184] Ibid.

[185] Adams, *Doctors in Blue*, 51–52.

[186] "Minutes of Executive Committee of the Scott County Soldiers' Relief Association," *Davenport Daily Gazette*, May 14, 1862, Morning edition, 1.

[187] Ira Gifford, "Letter from Ira Gifford," *Davenport Daily Gazette*, May 26, 1862, Morning edition, 1.

[188] Dr. Archibald Maxwell and Dr. Gamble, "Surgeons' Report," *Davenport Daily Gazette*, May 9, 1862, Morning edition, 3.

[189] Ibid.

[190] Ibid.

[191] Ibid.

[192] Ibid.

[193] Ibid.

[194] Newberry, *The U.S. Sanitary Commission in the Valley of the Mississippi*, 36.

[195] Grant, *Grant Memoirs,* 220–224.

[196] Ibid.

[197] Newberry, *The U.S. Sanitary Commission in the Valley of the Mississippi*, 40.

[198] Russell, Corresponding Secretary of the Scott County Soldiers' Relief Association, "The Surgical Committee," *Davenport Daily Gazette*, May 8, 1862, Morning edition, 1.

[199] A. S. Maxwell, "Letter to Mr. E. Russell dated May 7, 1862," *Davenport Daily Gazette*, May 14, 1862, 1.

[200] A. S. Maxwell, "Letter to Mr. E. Russell dated May 11, 1862, from the 8th Ward General Hospital at Hamburg Tennessee," *Davenport Daily Gazette*, May 19, 1862, 2.

[201] Ibid.

[202] Ira Gifford, "Letter to Reverend A. J. Kynett and Mr. Russell, dated May 19, 1862," *Davenport Daily Gazette*, May 26, 1862, 1.

[203] Ibid.

[204] A. S. Maxwell, "Letter to Mr. E. Russell dated May 11, 1862, from the 8th Ward General Hospital at Hamburg Tennessee," Davenport Daily Gazette, May 19, 1862, 2

[205] Ira Gifford, "Letter to Reverend A. J. Kynett and Mr. Russell, dated May 19, 1862," *Davenport Daily Gazette*, May 26, 1862, 1.

[206] Ibid.

[207] Ibid.

[208] Ibid.

[209] A. S. Maxwell, "Letter to Mr. E. Russell dated May 11, 1862, from the 8th Ward General Hospital at Hamburg Tennessee," Davenport Daily Gazette, May 19, 1862, 2

[210] Ira Gifford, "Letter to Reverend A. J. Kynett and Mr. Russell, dated May 19, 1862," *Davenport Daily Gazette*, May 26, 1862, 1

[211] A. S. Maxwell, "Letter to Mr. E. Russell dated May 11, 1862, from the 8th Ward General Hospital at Hamburg Tennessee," Davenport Daily Gazette, May 19, 1862, 2

[212] This is covered in a number of sources contemporary to that moment including the following articles and letters. L. C. Burwell, "Report of Mr. L. C. Burwell," *Davenport Daily Gazette*, June 5, 1862, Morning edition, 2. Letter from Dr. A. S. Maxwell to Governor Kirkwood, June 30, 1862, in Records of the Adjutant General, Sanitary Agents Reports, Civil War (series), State Historical Society of Iowa, Des Moines. A. S. Maxwell, "Letter to Mr. E. Russell," May 7, 1862," *Davenport Daily Gazette*, May 14, 1862, 1. A. S. Maxwell, "Letter to Mr. E. Russell," May 11, 1862, from the 8th Ward General Hospital at Hamburg, Tennessee," *Davenport Daily Gazette*, May 19, 1862, 2.

[213] Newberry, *The U.S. Sanitary Commission in the Valley of the Mississippi*, 43.

[214] Ibid, 42.

[215] Ibid, 40.

[216] Ibid.

[217] Ibid.

[218] Ibid, 42.

[219] Dr. Archibald S. Maxwell, "Letter to Reverend A. J. Kynett and Mr. Russell, dated May 19, 1862," *Davenport Daily Gazette*, May 26, 1862, 1.

[220] Executive Committee of the Scott County Soldiers' Relief Association, "Minutes of Meeting on May 7th", *The Davenport Daily Gazette*, May 14, 1862, 1.

[221] Dr. Archibald S. Maxwell, "Letter to Reverend A. J. Kynett and Mr. Russell, dated May 19, 1862," *Davenport Daily Gazette*, May 26, 1862, 1.

[222] Ibid.

[223] Letter from Dr. Archibald S. Maxwell to Governor Kirkwood, June 30, 1862, Records of the Adjutant General, Sanitary Agents Reports, Civil War (series), State Historical Society of Iowa, Des Moines.

[224] Letter from Assistant Surgeon 10th Iowa Volunteers and Approved by Lt. Col. Of the Regiment to Whom It May Concern, June 12, 1862, Records of the Adjutant General, Sanitary Agents Reports, Civil War (series), State Historical Society of Iowa, Des Moines.

[225] Ira Gifford, "State Agent at Pittsburg Landing", *Davenport Daily Gazette*, June 7, 1862, 1.

[226] Letter from Dr. A. S. Maxwell to Governor Kirkwood, June 30, 1862, Records of the Adjutant General, Sanitary Agents Reports, Civil War (series), State Historical Society of Iowa, Des Moines.

[227] Ibid.

[228] Editor, "Return of Dr. Maxwell," *Davenport Daily Gazette*, June 20, 1862, 1.

[229] Leonard, *Yankee Women*, 74, citing "Report of the Ladies Soldiers' Aid Society", *The Gate City*, April 15, 1862.

[230] Editor, "Minutes of Executive Committee, Scott County Soldiers' Relief Association," *Davenport Daily Gazette*, May 14, 1862, 1.

[231] Ibid.

[232] Ira Gifford, "Letter to Reverend A. J. Kynett and Mr. Russell, dated May 19, 1862," *Davenport Daily Gazette*, May 26, 1862, 1.

[233] Ibid.

[234] Letter to Governor Kirkwood from Reverend Kynett and several others, June 6, 1862, Records of Adjutant General, General Correspondence, Civil War (series), State Historical Society of Iowa, Des Moines.

[235] Letter from Hiram Price to Governor Kirkwood, June 30, 1862 Records of the Adjutant General, Sanitary Agents Reports, Civil War (series), State Historical Society of Iowa, Des Moines. Hiram Price wrote this note at the bottom of the Dr. Archibald S. Maxwell's report to Governor Kirkwood on the same date.

[236] Letter to Governor Kirkwood from Reverend Kynett and several others, June 6, 1862, Records of Adjutant General, General Correspondence, Civil War (series), State Historical Society of Iowa, Des Moines.

[237] Letter from Reverend Kynett to Governor Kirkwood, June 21, 1862, Records of Adjutant General, General Correspondence, Civil War (series), State Historical Society of Iowa, Des Moines.

[238] Letter from Hiram Price to Governor Kirkwood, June 30, 1862, Records of the Adjutant General, Sanitary Agents Reports, Civil War (series), State Historical Society of Iowa, Des Moines.

[239] "State Soldiers' Relief Convention," *Davenport Daily Gazette*, May 29, 1862.

[240] Ibid.

[241] Ibid.

[242] Ibid.

[243] Ibid.

[244] Ira Gifford, "Mr. Gifford's Report," *Davenport Daily Gazette*, July 1, 1862, 2.

[245] Editor, "Soldiers Aid Society Notice," *Davenport Daily Gazette*, July 3, 1862,1. Editor, "Arrival," *Davenport Daily Gazette*, July 3, 1862, 1.

[246] Editor, "Local Matters," *Davenport Daily Gazette*, July 4, 1862, 1.

[247] Ibid.

[248] Ibid.

[249] Ibid.

[250] Ibid.

[251] Ibid.

[252] Ibid.

[253] "Iowa Sanitary Association," *Burlington Weekly Hawk-Eye*, August 9, 1862, 2.

[254] Letter from Reverend Kynett to Governor Kirkwood, July 7, 1862, Records of Adjutant General, General Correspondence, Civil War (series), State Historical Society of Iowa, Des Moines.

[255] "Report of meeting of the ladies soldier's aid society and the Scott County Relief Association", *Davenport Daily Gazette*, July 7, 1862, 1.

[256] "The Governor at his home," *Davenport Daily Gazette*, July 8, 1862, 1.

[257] "Sheriff Sale," *Davenport Daily Gazette*, July 8, 1862, 1.

[258] Report of Ira Gifford to Governor Kirkwood concerning his activities from July 16, 1862 to November 1862,1, Records of the Adjutant General, Sanitary Agents Reports, Civil War (series), State Historical Society of Iowa, Des Moines. (Hereafter Gifford Report).

[259] Editor, "The Hospital Grounds—Another Inspection," *Davenport Daily Gazette*, July 12, 1862, 1.

[260] Letter from Ira Gifford to Annie Wittenmyer, July 12, 1862, Annie Turner Wittenmyer Papers 1861-1901, Special Collections, State Historical Society of Iowa, Des Moines; Gifford Report,1-3.

[261] Gifford Report, 1-3.

[262] Letter from Mr. Saunder to Governor Kirkwood, July 7, 1862, Records of Adjutant General, General Correspondence, Civil War (series), State Historical Society of Iowa, Des Moines.

[263] Adams, *Doctors in Blue*, 49.

[264] Letter from Ira Gifford to Governor Kirkwood, July 23, 1862, Records of Adjutant General, General Correspondence, Civil War (series), State Historical Society of Iowa, Des Moines.

[265] Adams, *Doctors in Blue*, 49.

[266] Letter from Ira Gifford to Governor Kirkwood, July 23, 1862, Records of Adjutant General, General Correspondence, Civil War (series), State Historical Society of Iowa, Des Moines.

[267] Gifford Report, 3

[268] Ibid; Letter from Ira Gifford to Annie Wittenmyer, July 26, 1862, written onboard the steamer G. W. Graham leaving Memphis, Tennessee, Annie Turner Wittenmyer Papers 1861-1901, Special Collections, State Historical Society of Iowa, Des Moines.

[269] Gifford Report, 3.

[270] Letter from Col. Ira Gifford to Mrs. Annie Wittenmyer, July 26, 1862, written onboard the steamer *G. W. Graham* leaving Memphis, Tennessee, Annie Turner Wittenmyer Papers 1861-1901, Special Collections, State Historical Society of Iowa, Des Moines.

[271] Ibid.

---

[272] Ibid.

[273] Letter from Col. Ira Gifford to Mrs. Annie Wittenmyer, July 22, 1862 written from the Everett House in St. Louis, Annie Turner Wittenmyer Papers 1861-1901, Special Collections, State Historical Society of Iowa, Des Moines.

[274] Gifford Report, 3.

[275] Adams, *Doctors in Blue*, 209.

[276] Letter from Col. Ira Gifford to Mrs. Annie Wittenmyer, July 26, 1862, written onboard the steamer *G. W. Graham* leaving Memphis, Annie Turner Wittenmyer Papers 1861-1901, Special Collections, State Historical Society of Iowa, Des Moines.

[277] Newberry, *The U.S. Sanitary Commission in the Valley of the Mississippi*, 43.

[278] Archibald Maxwell, "Letter from Dr. Maxwell," *Davenport Daily Gazette*, July 31, 1862, 1.

[279] Gifford Report, 4.

[280] Archibald Maxwell, "Letter from Dr. Maxwell," *Davenport Daily Gazette*, July 31, 1862, 1.

[281] Wittenmyer, *Under the Guns*, 135–136.

[282] Archibald Maxwell, "Letter from Dr. Maxwell," *Davenport Daily Gazette*, July 31, 1862, 1.

[283] Ibid.

[284] Letter from Col. Ira Gifford to Mrs. Annie Wittenmyer, dated July 26, 1862, written onboard the steamer *G. W. Graham* leaving Memphis, Tennessee, Annie Turner Wittenmyer Papers 1861-1901, Special Collections, State Historical Society of Iowa, Des Moines.

[285] Archibald Maxwell, "Letter from Dr. Maxwell," *Davenport Daily Gazette*, July 31, 1862, 1.

[286] Ibid.

[287] Gifford Report, 4; Letter from Col. Ira Gifford to Mrs. Annie Wittenmyer, dated July 26, 1862, written onboard the steamer *G. W. Graham* leaving Memphis, Tennessee, Annie Turner Wittenmyer Papers 1861-1901, Special Collections, State Historical Society of Iowa, Des Moines.

[288] Archibald Maxwell, "Letter from Dr. Maxwell," Davenport Daily Gazette, July 31, 1862, 1.

[289] Gifford Report, 6.

[290] Ibid.

[291] Gifford Report, 4; Letter from Col. Ira Gifford to Mrs. Annie Wittenmyer, dated July 26, 1862, written onboard the steamer *G. W. Graham* leaving Memphis, Tennessee, Annie Turner Wittenmyer Papers 1861-1901, Special Collections, State Historical Society of Iowa, Des Moines. This route was used by Colonel Gifford before him and seems the most plausible.

[292] Gifford Report, 6; Letter from Col. Ira Gifford to Mrs. Annie Wittenmyer, dated July 26, 1862, written onboard the steamer *G. W. Graham* leaving Memphis, Tennessee, Annie Turner Wittenmyer Papers 1861-1901, Special Collections, State Historical Society of Iowa, Des Moines.

[293] Gifford Report, 6.

[294] Ibid.

[295]Ibid; Dr. A. S. Maxwell, "August 11, 1862 Letter from Dr. Maxwell," *Davenport Daily Gazette*, August 16, 1862. The U.S. Sanitary Affairs Commission also extensively discusses its efforts to combat scurvy in the Western Armies. Newberry, *The U.S. Sanitary Commission in the Valley of the Mississippi,* 82–83.

[296] Dr. A. S. Maxwell, "August 11, 1862 Letter from Dr. Maxwell", *Davenport Daily Gazette*, August 16, 1862, 1.

[297] Ibid.

[298] Dr. A. S. Maxwell, "August 12, 1862 Letter from Dr. Maxwell", *Davenport Daily Gazette*, August 20, 1862, 1.

---

[299] Ibid.

[300] The two letters published on back to back days were as follows: Dr. A.S. Maxwell, "The Late Fights near Bolivar, Tenn. Letter from Dr. Maxwell, dated September 4, 1862", *Davenport Daily Gazette*, September 10, 1862, 1; Dr. A.S. Maxwell, "Letter from Dr. Maxwell, dated August 30, 1862", *Davenport Daily Gazette*, September 11, 1862, 2.

[301] Dr. A.S. Maxwell, "The Late Fights near Bolivar, Tenn. Letter from Dr. Maxwell, dated September 4, 1862", *Davenport Daily Gazette*, September 10, 1862, 1; Dr. A.S. Maxwell, "Letter from Dr. Maxwell, dated August 30, 1862", *Davenport Daily Gazette*, September 11, 1862, 2. This encounter was also mentioned by General Grant. Grant, *Grant's Memoir*, 237.

[302] Dr. A.S. Maxwell, "Letter from Dr. Maxwell, dated August 30, 1862", *Davenport Daily Gazette*, September 11, 1862, 2.

[303] Dr. A.S. Maxwell, "The Late Fights near Bolivar, Tenn. Letter from Dr. Maxwell, dated September 4, 1862", Davenport Daily Gazette, September 10, 1862, 1.

[304] Ibid.

[305] Letter from Ira Gifford to Annie Wittenmyer, August 16, 1862, Annie Turner Wittenmyer Papers 1861-1901, Special Collections, State Historical Society of Iowa, Des Moines. See also Gifford Report, 6.

[306] Letter from Ira Gifford to Annie Wittenmyer, August 21, 1862, Annie Turner Wittenmyer Papers 1861-1901, Special Collections, State Historical Society of Iowa, Des Moines.

[307] Ibid.

[308] "Extra Session of Legislature", *Davenport Daily Gazette*, August 20, 1862, 1.

[309] *Journal of the House of Representatives at the Extra Session of the Ninth General Assembly of the State of Iowa which convened at the Capital in Des Moines on Wednesday, the third day of September, A.D. 1862*, (Des Moines: F.W. Palmer, State Printer, 1862), 5.

---

[310] Letter from A.S. Maxwell to Annie Wittenmyer, dated August 27, 1862 (backside of letter from a different Surgeon to Annie Wittenmyer), Annie Turner Wittenmyer Papers 1861-1901, Special Collections, State Historical Society of Iowa, Des Moines.

[311] Ibid., 95. On September 11, 1862, the Senate informed the House that it had passed Senate File No. 37 which would eventually become Chapter 36. The Bill was read a first and second time. Representative Hardie attempted to refer it to committee but it failed. The rules were suspended to read it a third time and it did.

[312] *Acts and Resolutions Passed at the Extra Session of the Ninth General Assembly of the State of Iowa, which convened at the Capital, In Des Moines, on the third day of September, A.D. 1862* (Des Moines: F.W. Palmer, State Printer. 1862), 47.

[313] Grant, *Grant's Memoirs*, 241.

[314]Ibid; "The War News," *Davenport Daily Gazette*, September 24, 1862, 1.

[315] "Return of Col. Gifford," *Davenport Daily Gazette*, September 30, 1862, 1.

[316] Ibid.

[317] Letter from Archibald Maxwell to Annie Wittenmyer, September 25, 1862; Letter from John G. T. Holston, Medical Director of Dist. Of Tennessee, September 21, 1862, Annie Turner Wittenmyer Papers 1861-1901, Special Collections, State Historical Society of Iowa, Des Moines.

[318] *Biographical Dictionary of 1878*, 580.

[319] Letter from John G.T. Holston, Medical Director District of Tennessee to Governor Kirkwood, dated September 21, 1862, Records of Adjutant General, General Correspondence, Civil War (series), State Historical Society of Iowa, Des Moines.

[320] Letter from Surgeon for Iowa 11th Infantry Regiment, dated September 26, 1862, Records of Adjutant General, General Correspondence, Civil War (series), State Historical Society of Iowa, Des Moines.

[321] "Return of Col. Gifford," *Davenport Daily Gazette*, September 30, 1862, 1.

[322] Ibid.

[323] Cantwell, *A.S. Maxwell*, 138; *Biographical Dictionary of 1878*, 580.

[324] Letter from Augusta to her father, April 25, 1862, regarding the founding of Estes House. Letter available at State Historical Society of Iowa, Des Moines.

[325] Ira Gifford and Rev. A. J. Kynett, Report of Inspection of Keokuk Hospital to Governor Kirkwood, August 18, 1862, Records of Adjutant General, Sanitary Agents Reports, Civil War (series), State Historical Society of Iowa, Des Moines.

[326] Ira Gifford and Rev. A. J. Kynett , Report of Inspection of Keokuk Hospital to Governor Kirkwood, August 18, 1862, Records of Adjutant General, Sanitary Agents Reports, Civil War (series), State Historical Society of Iowa, Des Moines.

[327] Letter from Assistant Surgeon General Office in St. Louis to Dr. Archibald S. Maxwell, October 18, 1862; "Army Medical Intelligence," *American Medical Times*, Vol. 5 (July to December 1862), (Nov. 8, 1862), 264.

[328] Letter from Archibald S. Maxwell to Ira Gifford, October 16, 1862, Annie Turner Wittenmyer Papers 1861-1901, Special Collections, State Historical Society of Iowa, Des Moines.

[329] Letter from Archibald S. Maxwell to Ira Gifford, October 16, 1862, Annie Turner Wittenmyer Papers 1861-1901, Special Collections, State Historical Society of Iowa, Des Moines.; "For Keokuk and Corinth," *Daily Davenport Gazette*, October 18, 1862, 2.

[330] Archibald S. Maxwell, "From Keokuk Hospital," *Davenport Daily Gazette*, October 29, 1862, 2.

[331] "For Keokuk and Corinth," *Daily Davenport Gazette*, October 18, 1862, 2.

[332] Letter from Ira Gifford to Annie Wittenmyer, October 6, 1862, Annie Turner Wittenmyer Papers 1861-1901, Special Collections, State Historical Society of Iowa, Des Moines.

[333] Letter from A.S. Maxwell to Colonel Ira Gifford, October 16, 1862, Annie Turner Wittenmyer Papers 1861-1901, Special Collections, State Historical Society of Iowa, Des Moines. This letter was found in the Annie Turner Wittenmyer correspondence.

[334] Ibid.

[335] Ibid.

[336] Ibid.

[337] "Death of Dr. John F. Cook," *Holmes County Farmer*, February 2 1865, 3.

[338] Letter from A.S. Maxwell to Colonel Ira Gifford, October 16, 1862, Annie Turner Wittenmyer Papers 1861-1901, Special Collections, State Historical Society of Iowa, Des Moines.

[339] Archibald S. Maxwell, "From Keokuk Hospital," *Davenport Daily Gazette*, October 29, 1862, 2. "The Keokuk Hospital," *The Davenport Daily Gazette*, December 27, 1862, 4.

[340] Ira Gifford and Rev. A. J. Kynett , Report of Inspection of Keokuk Hospital to Governor Kirkwood, August 18, 1862, Records of Adjutant General, Sanitary Agents Reports, Civil War (series), State Historical Society of Iowa, Des Moines.

[341] Archibald S. Maxwell, "From Keokuk Hospital," *Davenport Daily Gazette*, October 29, 1862, 2. "A Boon to Iowa Soldiers," *Davenport Daily Gazette*, November 1, 1862, 4.

[342] Archibald S. Maxwell, "From Keokuk Hospital," *Davenport Daily Gazette*, October 29, 1862, 2.

[343] "A Boon to Iowa Soldiers," *Davenport Daily Gazette*, November 1, 1862, 4.

[344] Ira Gifford, "Letter from Col. I. M. Gifford," *Davenport Daily Gazette*, November 18, 1862, 1.

[345] "Our Sick at Keokuk," *Davenport Daily Gazette*, December 5, 1862, 1.

[346] Rev. P. P. Ingalls, Chaplain 3d Iowa Cavalry, "To the Aid Societies of Iowa," *Davenport Daily Gazette*, December 13, 1862, 2. The Letter was written on December 1, 1862, and sent from Helena, Arkansas.

[347] Ibid.

[348] Ibid.

[349] Ibid.

[350] Letter from Col. Ira Gifford to Annie Wittenmyer, October 31, 1862, Annie Turner Wittenmyer Papers 1861-1901, Special Collections, State Historical Society of Iowa, Des Moines.

[351] Rev. P. P. Ingalls, Chaplain 3d Iowa Cavalry, "To the Aid Societies of Iowa," Davenport Daily Gazette, December 13, 1862, 2.

[352] Ibid.

[353] Letter from Col. Ira Gifford to Annie Wittenmyer, October 31, 1862, Annie Turner Wittenmyer Papers 1861-1901, Special Collections, State Historical Society of Iowa, Des Moines.

[354] Ibid.

[355] Annie Wittenmyer, Iowa Sanitary Agent, "Sanitary Circular," *Burlington Weekly Hawk-Eye*, February 28, 1863, 2; Wittenmyer, Annie, Iowa Sanitary Agent, "Sanitary Circular," *Burlington Weekly Hawk-Eye*, March 14, 1863, 3.

[356] Newberry, *The U.S. Sanitary Commission in the Valley of the Mississippi*, 42–43; Adams, *Doctors in Blue*, 94.

[357] Adams, *Doctors in Blue*, 94.

[358] *Burlington Weekly Hawk-Eye*, May 30, 1863, 6.

[359] Forman, *The Western Sanitary Commission*, 74–75.

[360] Ibid.

[361] Annie Wittenmyer, Iowa Sanitary Agent, "Sanitary Circular," *Burlington Weekly Hawk-Eye*, March 14, 1863, 3.

[362] Annie Wittenmyer, Iowa Sanitary Agent, "Sanitary Circular," *Cedar Falls Gazette*, March 13, 1863, 2.

---

[363] Reverend A. J. Kynett, "Sanitary Circular 11 from the Iowa Army Sanitary Commission," *Burlington Weekly Hawk-Eye*, 6 (Saturday March 28, 1863)(Burlington, Iowa).

[364] A. Wittenmyer, "Circular From Mrs. Wittenmyer to the Soldiers Aid Societies of Iowa," *Burlington Weekly Hawk Eye*, June 13, 1863, 8.

[365] Ibid.

[366] Ibid.

[367] Letter from Dr. Archibald S. Maxwell to Annie Wittenmyer, dated April 12, 1863, Annie Turner Wittenmyer Papers 1861-1901, Special Collections, State Historical Society of Iowa, Des Moines.

[368] Ibid.

[369] Ibid.

[370] Ibid.

[371] Theresa R. McDevitt, "'A Melody Before Unknown': the Civil War Experiences of Mary and Amanda Shelton," *The Annals of Iowa*, V. 63 Number 2, 109. (State Historical Society of Iowa Spring 2004).

[372] Letter from Dr. Archibald S. Maxwell to Mrs. Annie Wittenmyer, May 20, 1863, Annie Turner Wittenmyer Papers 1861-1901, Special Collections, State Historical Society of Iowa, Des Moines.

[373] Newberry, *The U.S. Sanitary Commission in the Valley of the Mississippi*, 93.

[374]Letter from Dr. Archibald S. Maxwell to Mrs. Annie Wittenmyer, May 20, 1863, Annie Turner Wittenmyer Papers 1861-1901, Special Collections, State Historical Society of Iowa, Des Moines.

[375] Letter from Dr. Archibald S. Maxwell to Mrs. Annie Wittenmyer, June 8, 1863, Annie Turner Wittenmyer Papers 1861-1901, Special Collections, State Historical Society of Iowa, Des Moines.

[376] Ibid.

[377] Ibid.

[378] Ibid.

[379] Transport Order for Annie Wittenmyer and Dr. Maxwell, June 23, 1863, Maxwell Family Archives.

[380] Wittenmyer, *Under the Guns*, 139.

[381] Ibid.

[382] Ibid.138-139.

[383] Ibid., 147–149.

[384] Ibid., 147–149.

[385] Ibid.

[386] Ibid., 187.

[387] Ibid., 187.

[388] Ibid at 174; Letter from Dr. Archibald S. Maxwell to Mrs. Annie Wittenmyer, August 19, 1863, Annie Turner Wittenmyer Papers 1861-1901, Special Collections, State Historical Society of Iowa, Des Moines..

[389] Maxwell, A. Dr. and Wittenmyer, Annie, State Sanitary Agents, Sanitary Circular, July 30, 1863. (Iowa State Historical Society Collections).

[390] Ibid.

[391] Forman, *The Western Sanitary Commission*, 72.

[392] Ibid. Newberry, *The U.S. Sanitary Commission in the Valley of the Mississippi*, 82; Stille, *History of United States Sanitary Commission,* 320. The addressing the problems with Scurvy and the Commission's efforts to address it.

[393] Letter from Annie Wittenmyer to Archibald S. Maxwell, August 3, 1863, Annie Turner Wittenmyer Papers 1861-1901, Special Collections, State Historical Society of Iowa, Des Moines.

[394] Map of the Vicksburg Siege Lines, Records of the Adjutant General, Sanitary Agents Reports, Civil War (series), State Historical Society of Iowa, Des Moines.

[395] Letter from E. J. Mathis to Annie Wittenmyer, August 4, 1863, Annie Turner Wittenmyer Papers 1861-1901, Special Collections, State Historical Society of Iowa, Des Moines.

[396] Letter from Annie Wittenmyer to Dr. Archibald S. Maxwell, August 3, 1863, Annie Turner Wittenmyer Papers 1861-1901, Special Collections, State Historical Society of Iowa, Des Moines.

[397] Letter from Annie Wittenmyer to Dr. Archibald S. Maxwell, August 3, 1863, Annie Turner Wittenmyer Papers 1861-1901, Special Collections, State Historical Society of Iowa, Des Moines.

[398] Ibid.

[399] Iowa Sanitary Commission, *Report of the Iowa Sanitary Commission from Its Organization October 13, 1861 to the Close of Its Service By the Transfer of Its Work to the New Commission December 1, 1863 To His Excellency Samuel J. Kirkwood, Governor of Iowa* (Davenport: Publishing House of Luse, Lane & Co.,1864), 10

[400] Ibid.

[401] Letter from Archibald S. Maxwell to Mrs. Annie Wittenmyer, August 19, 1863, Annie Turner Wittenmyer Papers 1861-1901, Special Collections, State Historical Society of Iowa, Des Moines.

[402] Ibid.

[403] Ibid.

[404] Ibid.

[405] Letter from Annie Wittenmyer to Governor Kirkwood, December 18, 1863, Samuel J. Kirkwood Papers 1841-1894, Special Collections, State Historical Society of Iowa, Des Moines.

[406] Letter from Archibald S. Maxwell to Mrs. Annie Wittenmyer, August 19, 1863, Annie Turner Wittenmyer Papers 1861-1901, Special Collections, State Historical Society of Iowa, Des Moines.

[407] Ibid.

[408] Maxwell, A. Dr. and Wittenmyer, Annie, State Sanitary Agents, Sanitary Circular, July 30, 1863. (Iowa State Historical Society Collections).

[409]Letter from Dr. A. S. Maxwell to Adjutant General of Iowa N. Baker, October 8, 1863, Records of the Adjutant General, Sanitary Agents Reports, Civil War (series), State Historical Society of Iowa, Des Moines.

[410] Ibid.

[411] Grant, *Grant Memoirs*, 340. General Grant offers an interesting discussion of the break-up of the Army used to take Vicksburg. As he does throughout his book, he detailed strategies and avenues not used. In particular he discusses the failure to use that Army to attack Mobile, Alabama, which Grant claimed could have caused Bragg to retreat from Chattanooga, Tennessee.

[412] Ibid.

[413] Ibid.

[414] Dr. Archibald S. Maxwell, Report to Governor Kirkwood, November 6, 1863, Records of the Adjutant General, Sanitary Agents Reports, Civil War (series), State Historical Society of Iowa, Des Moines (hereafter the "November 6th Report").

[415] Adams, *Doctors in Blue*, 199–200.

[416] Adams, *Doctors in Blue*, 146.

[417] M. Goldsmith, Surgeon U.S.V. Superintendent of Hospitals at Louisville, Kentucky, "Bromine as a Prophylactic," *The American Medical Times, Being a Weekly Series of the New York Journal of Medicine*, Vol. VI January to July 1863, Stephen Smith M.D. Geo. Shrady M.D Eds., 141: Adams, *Doctors in Blue*, 146.

[418] Letter from Dr. A.S. Maxwell to Mrs. Annie Wittenmyer, dated October 19, 1863, Annie Turner Wittenmyer Papers 1861-1901, Special Collections, State Historical Society of Iowa, Des Moines.

[419] November 6th Report.

[420] Letter from Dr. Archibald S. Maxwell to Mrs. Annie Wittenmyer, October 28, 1863, Annie Turner Wittenmyer Papers 1861-1901, Special Collections, State Historical Society of Iowa, Des Moines.

[421] Ibid.

[422] Wittenmyer, *Under the Guns*, 187.

[423] November 6th Report.

[424] Ibid.

[425] Ibid.

[426] Undated Letter from Dr. Archibald S. Maxwell with accompanying letter from Colonel of 8th Iowa Infantry enclosed with November 6th Report.

[427] Dr. Archibald S. Maxwell, Iowa State Sanitary Agent, Report to N.B. Baker, Adjutant General and Quartermaster, State of Iowa, November 6, 1863, from Vicksburg, Mississippi, Hospital Correspondence, State of Iowa Historical Archives.

[428] Ibid.

[429] Ibid.

[430] Ibid.

[431] Dr. Archibald S. Maxwell, Iowa State Sanitary Agent, Report to N. B. Baker, Adjutant General and Quartermaster, State of Iowa, December 9, 1863, from Vicksburg, Mississippi, Hospital Correspondence, State of Iowa Historical Archives. This report reappears in the 1863 Report of the Adjutant General and Acting Quarter Master without Dr. Maxwell's statistics. It can be found at Dr. Archibald S. Maxwell, "Dr. Maxwell's Report," *Report of the Adjutant General and Acting Quartermaster*

General of the State of Iowa January 1, 1863 to January 11, 1864 (Des Moines: F.W. Palmer, State Printer, 1864), 765–767. (Also referred to as December 9th Report).

[432] Ibid, 765.

[433] Ibid.

[434] Ibid.

[435] Ibid.

[436] Ibid.

[437] Ibid, 766.

[438] Ibid.

[439] Ibid.

[440] Ibid.

[441] Ibid.

[442] Ibid.

[443] Letter from Dr. Archibald S. Maxwell to N. B. Baker, Adjutant General and Quartermaster, State of Iowa, December 10, 1863, from Vicksburg, Mississippi, Records of Adjutant General, Sanitary Agents Reports, Civil War (series), State Historical Society of Iowa, Des Moines.

[444] Ibid.

[445] *Biographical Dictionary of 1878*, 580.

[446] "The Sanitary Convention," *Burlington Weekly Hawk-Eye*, November 21, 1863, 1. (reprint from *Gate City*).

[447] "Vindication of Mrs. Wittenmyer," *Burlington Weekly Hawk-Eye*, November 28, 1863, 4.

[448] "Iowa State Sanitary Commission," *Cedar Falls Gazette*, November 27, 1863, 2.

[449] Ibid.

[450] *Biographical Dictionary of 1878*, 581.

[451] "The Sanitary Leaders," *Cedar Falls Gazette*, December 18, 1863, 3.

[452] "The War on Annie Wittenmyer," *Cedar Falls Gazette*, April 1, 1864, 2.

[453] *Journal of the House of Representatives of the Tenth General Assembly of the State of Iowa, Which Convened at the Capital in Des Moines, January 11, 1864* (Des Moines: F.W. Palmer, State Printer, 1864), 35–36.

[454] Ibid.

[455] Ibid.

[456] Letter from Reverend Kynett to Governor Kirkwood, December 9, 1863, Samuel J. Kirkwood Papers 1841-1894, Special Collections, State Historical Society of Iowa, Des Moines.

[457] Letter from Reverend Kynett to Governor Kirkwood, December 29, 1863, Samuel J. Kirkwood Papers 1841-1894, Special Collections, State Historical Society of Iowa, Des Moines.

[458] *Journal of the Senate of the Tenth General Assembly of the State of Iowa, Which Convened at the Capital in Des Moines, January 11, 1864*, (Des Moines: F.W. Palmer, State Printer, 1864), 199–200.

[459] Ibid.

[460] *Journal of the House of Representatives of the Tenth General Assembly of the State of Iowa*, 236–237.

[461] Ibid.

[462] Ibid.

[463] Ibid., 274–275.

[464] Ibid., 277.

[465] Ibid.

[466] Ibid., 342.

[467] Ibid., 492.

[468] Ibid., 545.

[469] Ibid., 350.

[470] Ibid., 648.

[471] *Biographical Dictionary of 1878*, 581.

[472] Ibid.

[473] Ibid.

[474] "Advertisement," *Davenport Daily Gazette*, June 25, 1866, 2.

[475] Cantwell, *A.S. Maxwell*, 138.

[476] "Income Returns for 1865," *Davenport Daily Gazette*, July 19, 1866, 4. Everyone's amounts were reported in the newspaper on which taxes were paid. $600 and other items exempted by law were deducted from the amounts.

[477] Edward Russell, ed., "Our Fellow Citizen Dr. Maxwell," *Davenport Daily Gazette*, May 30, 1867, 2.

[478] "Meeting of the Board of Health," *Davenport Daily Gazette*, August 24, 1866, 4.

[479] "Medical Society," *Davenport Daily Gazette*, May 11, 1866, 4. *Biographical Dictionary of 1878*, 580.

[480] Cantwell, *A.S. Maxwell*, 139.

[481] United States House of Representatives, 43d Congress, 2nd Session, *The Cholera Epidemic of 1873 in the United States*, Ex. Doc. No. 95, Washington D.C., Government Printing Office, 1875, 456-457.

[482] Ibid.

[483] Ibid.

[484] Ibid.

[485] I am the great-great grandson of George Bancroft Maxwell. George Bancroft had a medical practice in Scott County, Iowa. George Bancroft had several children. My genealogy is beyond the scope of this book.

[486] November 6th Report and December 9th Report.

[487] For a list of translations from Latin of the medicines in the medical list, see www.medicalantiques.com/civilwar.